DETOX 101

DETOX 101

A 21-Day Guide to Cleansing Your Body
through Juicing, Exercise, and Healthy Living

Jessi Andricks

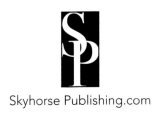

Skyhorse Publishing.com

Skyhorse Publishing books may be purchased in bulk at special discounts for sales promotion, corporate gifts, fund-raising, or educational purposes. Special editions can also be created to specifications. For details, contact the Special Sales Department, Skyhorse Publishing, 307 West 36th Street, 11th Floor, New York, NY 10018 or info@skyhorsepublishing.com.

Skyhorse® and Skyhorse Publishing® are registered trademarks of Skyhorse Publishing, Inc.®, a Delaware corporation.

Visit our website at www.skyhorsepublishing.com.

10 9 8 7 6 5 4 3 2 1

Library of Congress Cataloging-in-Publication Data is available on file.

Cover design by Owen Corrigan
Cover photo credit Thinkstock

Print ISBN: 978-1-62914-717-8
Ebook ISBN: 978-1-62914-916-5

Printed in China

Table of Contents:

Introduction

For years, I suffered from digestive issues. Painful stomach cramps, bloating, gas, constipation, diarrhea, and even the occasional heartburn. But I always thought it was normal, that this was how most people lived too. The sad part is that it's true. Most people suffer from one or all of these symptoms on a daily basis, sometimes without even realizing it.

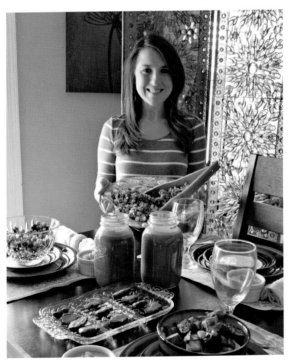

In my twenties, my symptoms became worse and I learned that I suffered from lactose intolerance, which means that I cannot properly digest the lactose, or sugar, in cow's milk due to a decrease in lactase enzymes needed to digest it. I grew up eating cheese and yogurt, and drinking milk every night at dinner, but suddenly my system was revolting against it.

I cut out the dairy and started looking for alternatives. I tried lactose free milk and eventually soy milk. In researching alternatives, I started to learn more about all-natural and organic foods, which were suddenly becoming more and more mainstream. This was the beginning of completely changing my diet from the Standard American "Healthy" Diet to a truly healthy, holistic diet.

From there, I kept researching more, changed my exercise habits, completely changed my eating habits, and learned to live a life around my passion—holistic living. I started practicing yoga and immediately fell in love with the way it made me feel physically and mentally. After practicing for a few years, I became certified to teach yoga and group fitness, and I even developed an energizing blend of classes to increase energy as you work out, which I called Energy Flow. After helping people become physically healthier through exercise, I made the step to helping people with their diets as a health coach. These practices have given me the unique tools to help others live healthier lives through better food awareness, functional fitness, and stress-reducing daily activities.

Years after changing my diet, career, and fitness outlook, I began to notice some digestive troubles again. I wasn't sure what was causing them, so I decided to try a cleanse. It happened to be a new year, I had just completed my first race, and I was in the process of changing my career. It seemed like the perfect time to recharge and cleanse the old patterns, habits, and foods out of my system.

The cleanse was simple: juice, mostly raw, no gluten, sugar, meat, dairy, or eggs. No alcohol or caffeine (except green tea). The idea was to eliminate food allergen triggers and reduce inflammation. This was when I realized that cutting out wheat stopped my stomach pains again. I used this as an elimination diet, to see what would hurt my stomach and how I could make it better, but it also ended up changing my diet even more.

Before the cleanse, I had become vegetarian, ate mostly local and organic foods, and occasionally had goat milk (lactose isn't in it), yogurt, and seafood. I would start my day with oatmeal and end up hungry soon after. But during the cleanse, I juiced every morning with 50 percent raw foods and never once felt deprived. I felt more energized, had less digestive pains, and felt that I was learning to heal my own dietary troubles and bring more awareness into what I was eating.

I now continue to juice or have smoothies everyday for breakfast and I finally feel full through the morning. I drink tea because I enjoy the flavors and not for a caffeine buzz. And overall, I feel healthier, more aware, and better connected to my own health.

And now it's your turn.

In the next twenty-one days, you will learn to juice, reduce inflammation, clean out your digestive tract, and regain energy not only through food but also through mind-body exercise, positive daily mottos, and easy meditations. All to help you live a healthy, happy life.

Chapter One:
Overview of Detox

CLEANSING

WHAT IS A CLEANSE?

Cleansing. Just the thought of it might be enough for you to close this book and never come back. But keep reading. I promise you can do it.

The truth is, a cleanse doesn't have to be a big scary affair. Cleanses don't have to be all consuming. You don't have to live in a retreat center or a cabin in the woods, only consuming lemon water and syrup for days on end. You can live in the real world, eat real food, and still detox your body and mind from all the junk that has been stored up over time.

When you cleanse, you consume simple, pure foods and drinks. These become your detox ninjas. They fight their ways through your body and cut through the garbage. You release toxins, fat, and build up in your digestive tract. Your body begins to glow from the inside out. And you feel fresh and new. *That* is what a cleanse is all about. There are many types of cleanse, and they can range from more restrictive to simply eating less processed foods and more

vegetables. Whatever the type or intensity of the cleanse, they are all designed to help you recharge your system and make healthy changes that last well beyond your detox program.

WHY DO WE CLEANSE?

Whether you are a health nut or a junk food lover, a detox program may be needed in your diet from time to time.

A cleanse or detox program is simply a time to let to your digestive system rest, to clear out some clutter that may have built up inside, and to refresh your body, mind, and spirit. You'll release toxins that have built up in your system and flush them out, leaving you more energized and less bogged down. The less buildup you have in your system, the less your body has to work in overdrive to clean up the messes within your system. Constantly eating foods that block your energy and digestion, stressing and thinking negative thoughts, and living a sedentary lifestyle all lead to excess toxins in the body and poorly functioning organs and digestion.

When you detox, you start to break down some of these toxins, flushing them out of your system. As they release and you add more energizing, fresh, and healthy foods to your diet, as well as exercising more, you start to recharge your digestive tract, improve the function of your body, and release built-up stress. The more energy you have, the better you feel and the more likely you are to stick with these practices well beyond the detoxification process.

A cleanse is not a quick fix for disease or weight loss. It isn't guaranteed to help you drop twenty pounds a week or reverse any medical conditions. A cleanse is just the beginning steps on your journey to a healthier, happier, more vibrant you. You just might find a newer, fresher outlook on life when you tune in, change your diet, and take care of yourself.

HOW DO WE CLEANSE?

Cleansing and detoxing are easy to do. You take away certain parts of what you eat and focus instead on eating and drinking things that will help support your system. It is all about cleaning up your body from the inside out and letting go of the toxins that are triggering poor health and digestion.

A real cleanse means you cut out some of the food that may be triggering indigestion. These usually include dairy, wheat/gluten, some soy, caffeine, sugar, alcohol, eggs, meat, and, most importantly, processed foods. The list may seem depriving at first, but soon you'll start to notice all of the other foods that are available to you. These foods are high in nutrients and low in toxic chemicals and digestive irritants. When your body starts to eat these on a regular basis, you begin to crave the high quality of fruits, vegetables, seeds, nuts, and gluten-free grains. During your cleanse, you'll learn to add in foods, drinks, and herbs that kick-start your digestion. You'll start to feel better, healthier, and full of energy.

Cleansing and detoxing are really much simpler than they seem. They don't have to be a drastic, unrealistic way of eating, exercising, and living. Detoxes are really just simple things that help you get back to a healthy, happy state through reworking your approach to what you eat and drink, how you move, and why you think what you think. You start out as a minimalist and steadily build your way back to a regular diet, you exercise at an energizing pace, and you get back to positive thinking about who you are and what you feel. You get back to who you really are and how you want your life to be, only now you've made *big* changes—changes that make you love your life and want to stay vibrant and healthy.

Chapter Two:
Digestion 101

POOP AND DIGESTION: WHERE DETOX BEGINS AND ENDS

Good digestion is the key to good health. Poor digestion is a path straight into poor health. When you are digesting food and drinks efficiently, your body is collecting the nutrients from your foods and processing out the rest. It's that "rest" that we eliminate via excretion, a.k.a. pooping. This elimination process helps us to get rid of the waste and toxins that our organs have sorted through and sent onward to be removed from our systems.

When you have good digestion, you are free from painful bloating, gas, and diarrhea or constipation. You have regular bowel movements one to three times each day to eliminate the excess from what you have eaten, and these are strain free and, well, smooth. You also feel lighter from the inside out, your skin tone is brighter, and you feel more energized. This is because you body is receiving all of the goodness that it needs to function at the optimal level. And it is receiving all of this from purely good food and exercise.

When you have poor digestion, a few things start to happen. First, you start to have poor breakdown of the foods we eat. When you are unable to fully chew or your stomach doesn't break down your foods, your body isn't able to absorb all of the nutrients in your foods. When you can't absorb your nutrients, you end up needing to take supplements or eat *more* food just to maintain the proper amount of vitamins and minerals.

Poor digestion also means that the toxins stay in your body for a longer amount of time. Once your organs start to assimilate the nutrients and release the toxins from your foods, they are collected together in your large intestines. When your digestive system is working properly, you are able to release this in the form of a bowel movement. When you are constipated or even just pooping less than once a day, these toxins sit in your system and you start to reabsorb them, starting the whole cycle over again. With better

3

digestion, you remove these toxins from your body rather than re-circulate them, and you end up with better overall health.

To improve your digestion, you can eat certain foods including healthy fruits, vegetables, and high-fiber foods, drink more water to keep flushing out your digestive tract, use herbs and digestive enzymes to increase the effectiveness of your food, and exercise to help push things along; but doing all of this at once can overwhelm your system and possibly even lead to gas, bloating, and discomfort. This is where a cleanse, and specifically juicing, comes in handy.

JUICING 101

Chances are your digestive system has been working overtime to try to extract any possible nutrition from the junk that we put in our bodies. Overtime, all of the processed, overcooked, and nutritionally devoid foods get built up in your system. This might take the form of constipation, literally building up in your system, or it might show up as sluggishness, tiredness, stomach aches, or poor immunity. Whatever it is, these foods leave behind physical debris in your digestive tract, leave toxins in your bloodstream and organs, and cause you to work overtime to help digest and clean them out. When you cleanse, it's your chance to give your digestive system a break, clean it out, and recharge it. This is where juicing comes in.

Juicing is a very important part of good health and digestion. When you juice a fruit or vegetable, you are extracting all the natural liquid, nutrients, and enzymes from them, while at the same time removing the fiber. Fiber is good for you and is indeed an essential part of your diet, but it requires a great deal of effort to digest and push through your system. All the time spent digesting fiber leads to less time digesting your nutrients and enzymes. With fresh juice, you have removed the fiber, so you are able to immediately start digesting the enzymes and flushing out your system. Smoothies are a great choice as well, since the blending breaks down the fiber, allowing you to absorb the enzymes quickly. Since the fiber is in them still, though, they are much heavier than juice and are a little harder on your system to digest. They are great for a day when you know that a juice just isn't going to sustain you until your next meal/snack.

Since your juice and smoothies are already broken down for you, the nutrients within them are more easily available to absorb directly into your system with much less effort. These nutrients and enzymes work to replenish your organs, especially your liver and kidneys, which filter toxins away from your bloodstream and out of your system. When you juice, you are giving your organs a straight shot of nutrition to keep you *and* your organs working at an optimal level. This helps to improve your overall digestion, in both the quality and quantity of what you receive from your foods.

In this program, juicing takes center stage as a healer and recharger for your body, mind, and spirit. It will be used to detox and cleanse your system, give you more energy, and help you ease any aches and pains in your digestive tract or energy levels that might be causing you stress. You'll be juicing or blending smoothies at least once a day in the morning, and you may even sneak some in throughout the day as snacks and with meals. You'll replenish your system after eight long hours of sleep with a healthy dose of digestive and cleansing enzymes to get you feeling refreshed and energized.

ACIDITY:

One piece of the food puzzle to take into account when you start to eat healthy, and especially when you are on a cleanse, is acidity. This is the amount of acid and alkalinity in your bloodstream, or your pH level. Some foods are more acidic than others from the start, and when you ingest them they lead to an increase in the acidity level in your body. There are also some alkaline (less acidic) foods that become acidic once you eat them, which in turn can increase the acidity level of your body.

So what's the big deal with being acidic?

Our bodies like to perform at their optimal level, leading to better health and less stress internally. That optimum level is at a balanced alkaline pH level of 7.4 and will fight to get back to this level, stressing your organs as they try to restore balance and pulling calcium out of your bones to reduce the acidity level. When we are close to this balanced pH level, our bodily systems function with ease and we are able to use our energy to digest and absorb nutrients rather than use it to fight against an acidic bloodstream.

Most of the time, we are shifted slightly into the more acidic side of the scale, which can lead to inflammation. Inflammation occurs naturally in the body as a response to injuries and disease. When you get a bug bite or a scrape and your skin swells, this is inflammation doing its job to send antibodies to the source and heal it. When we stay in an acidic state, our bodies are constantly trying to repair the damage, working in overdrive. This inflammation turns on a fight response in our cells and sends the body into overdrive, leaving you fatigued, stressed, and weak. This can lead to a host of diseases in the bodies as your immune system weakens, including cancer, heart disease, diabetes, and even obesity.

The most acidic foods are meat, dairy, wheat, alcohol, caffeine, and some citrus foods—not lemons, though, they actually turn alkaline once in your body. These cause you to shift away from the balanced 7.4 pH level toward a more acidic level. By avoiding these foods, especially when you are trying to remove toxins from your system, you are helping your system come to a more balanced and optimally functioning state.

There are also some lifestyle habits that can also contribute to acidity. Drinking and smoking are big health no-no's and cause acidic conditions in the body, but so do certain seemingly healthy habits, such as too much exercise and too much stress.

Exercising too hard can cause your body to overheat and become overworked. When this happens, your muscles and tissues become inflamed and your pH level turns acidic. It also zaps your energy, because you are internally spending so much time repairing and recharging your sywstems. Instead, exercising efficiently and functionally, without pushing too far passed your edge, can help you reduce acidity, inflammation, and stress. Stress itself is a big inflammation trigger. When you are stressed, you automatically tap into your flight or fight response and your body, particularly your adrenals, go into overdrive to help calm your nervous system. You heart rate rises, your brain feels frazzled, your stomach feels tied in knots, and your blood feels like it is boiling. All of these are your body signaling a major breakdown and a major stressful event. Your adrenal glands work to help even this out and can become fatigued and overrun, leading to a permanent feeling of stress. While your body tries to compensate for this, the acidic condition rises and your pH gets thrown off, making you more susceptible to disease.

When we eat healthy, exercise in tune with our bodies, and meditate to clear stress, we help reduce acidity, prevent disease, and clear out the toxic build-up in our bodies, mind, and spirit that keep us from feeling happy, healthy, and alive.

FOODS

ORGANIC IS KING

There is no way to get around it. Food that is grown in rich soil, without poisonous pesticides, herbicides, or GMOs, is the best food for you. These foods are pure, straight from the earth, and full of goodness. They are commonly referred to as organic. Organic simply means that the foods were grown without any conventional pesticides or herbicides from spray, soil, or in the seeds themselves. Certified organic foods have strict guidelines the farmers have to maintain in order to stay certified. There are also local farmers that can't afford to pay for the certification but use the same processes when they grow their crops. When you eat organically, you know you are eating free of chemicals and added toxins that will be stored up and put stress on your internal systems.

Organic foods, especially your produce, are an important part of everyday health, but they are especially important to any detox program. When you eat foods that are grown with toxic sprays and seeds, no matter how much you scrub your food, traces of these chemicals will be contained within the food and, therefore, within your system. When you eat mostly organic, you are helping to reduce the amount of toxic pesticides going into your system, so your body doesn't have to work overtime to clear them back out.

Dirty Dozen: The Most Toxic Nonorganic Produce	Clean Fifteen: The Least Toxic Nonorganic Produce
• Peaches • Apples • Sweet Bell Peppers • Celery • Nectarines • Strawberries • Cherries • Pears • Grapes (Imported) • Spinach • Lettuce • Potatoes	• Onions • Sweet corn • Pineapples • Avocado • Cabbage • Sweet peas • Asparagus • Mangoes • Eggplant • Kiwi • Cantaloupe (domestic) • Sweet potatoes • Grapefruit • Papayas • Mushrooms

As you are detoxing, you want to make sure you are adding as *little* toxins as possible into your system. Much of these come into your body through what you breathe in and what you eat or drink. Unfortunately, we can't always control our air quality. What we can control is the amount of toxins we receive via our foods. Choose fresh foods that are high in quality and low in toxins whenever possible. Shop at health food stores, your local grocer, or through farmers markets and local farmers to find the best price and quality. If you can't afford all organic or you have limited availability in your area, here is the list of the cleanest and meanest when it comes to pesticides.

EAT YOUR GREENS

Cruciferous vegetables, also known as leafy greens, are also an essential part of your detox program. These include vegetables such as kale, spinach, broccoli, collards, turnip greens, and all lettuces. Leafy greens have the most nutrients per bite than any other food group, which means that each bite of these greens has more vitamins and minerals per bite than any other food. Basically you get more bang for your bite. They also tend to be low on calories but high on fiber, and even protein, so you can eat a lot, feel full, and consume less calories. They are also full of chlorophyll, which gives them their green color. The chlorophyll is a byproduct of photosynthesis (a.k.a. plant food and energy from the sun) and is both cleansing and energizing when consumed. Leafy greens will be included with each meal throughout the three weeks, including breakfast. Greens will become the base of your smoothies and juices as well as the main stage in your salads and entrees, giving you a multitude of nutrients, enzymes, fiber, protein, chlorophyll, and flavor. They will keep you feeling full, help curb cravings, and help you get healthy, clean, and energized naturally. Remember to keep these organic whenever possible, since you will be consuming a large amount of these in the next few weeks.

LIFESTYLE

EXERCISE

An integral part of staying healthy is moving your body, a.k.a. exercise. There is no way around it; to stay healthy and have your body function at its maximum ability, you've got to get up and move, specifically in a way that builds strength, burns away excess, and releases tension and toxins. This movement helps to keep your muscles strong, keeps you limber, and even tones your organs, improving their function. When your organs are strong, they function more efficiently and are able to do their job with less effort. When your digestive system muscles are strong, you are better able to push toxins out of your system, flushing your body and keeping your digestive tract regular.

The main key to exercising during a cleanse is to keep it simple. Focus on simply moving, releasing, and re-energizing. Exercising too much and too intensely can cause strain and stress on the body, which creates inflammation and acidity. These both leave your body working in overdrive to bring you back to a balanced state and replenish your systems. You'll feel tired, sluggish, and zapped of energy. Instead, focus on moving with awareness of how you feel and exercising to create *more* energy in your body. In the case of exercise, sometimes less really is more.

Each day, you'll take forty-five to seventy-five minutes to move your body in some way. Some days it will be strengthening, some days it will be more cardio, and some days you will simply stretch to release tension and stress. Carve out time each day to commit to your exercise. If you can, make it the same time each day and start to get yourself into a routine that you'll be more likely to stick with during and after the program. You'll help aid in digestion as well as improve your overall muscle tone, weight loss, and even your skin tone.

SLEEP

Sleep is important. In fact, it is one of the most important things you can do to stay healthy, but it is also one of the easiest things to push aside. Life gets hectic, your schedule gets busy, and you start to burn the candle at both ends. You stay up too late, get up too early, and live in a sleep deprived state most of the time.

When you are sleep deprived, both your mind and your body suffer. Sleep is when your body repairs and heals itself from all of the wear and tear it endures during the day. When you sleep, your cells replenish you and help you to maintain a healthy, happy lifestyle. Sleep deprivation leads to higher stress levels and a lower ability to handle stress due to all of your systems constantly working to try to regain balance and restore their vitality. When this happens, your body is signaled to release stress-fighting hormones, which taxes out your adrenal system, making it hard for you to handle stress both mentally and physically. Because of this breakdown in your defenses, it can lead to weight gain, high blood pressure, and anxiety, among a host of other health problems. Sleep deprivation also makes you less alert and minimizes your abilities to make good decisions regarding your health. When you are tired, it is much more likely that you reach for sugary, processed foods and caffeine to give you an extra rush of energy, which will only lead to a crash later on. Convenience foods start to seem more appealing, because you are too tired to plan a meal and spend the time preparing it. You may notice you exercise less, because you feel too depleted to workout, which in turn wreaks havoc on your digestive system.

This added sugar and caffeine, lack of movement, and digestive upset can lead to bloating, weight gain, and further depleted energy levels.

To help improve or maintain a healthy sleep schedule, make sure you get approximately eight hours of sleep each night. Avoid caffeine later in the afternoons or evenings, so it won't still be in your system when you go to bed. Try not to go to bed hungry or super full from your meals, as this might disrupt your digestion and keep you up during the night. Step away from your computer or television a few minutes before you decide to head to bed, so your body and mind are less stimulated and it is easier to fall asleep. Make it a point to wind down before bed with a few yoga stretches, a breathing exercise, or a quick meditation to help calm your body and mind and prepare them for a good night's sleep. If you need extra help falling asleep, try some chamomile tea, relaxing music, lavender-scented candles, or a few more deep stretches.

THE TRIFECTA: MEDITATION, BREATH WORK, AND JOURNALING

This can often seem like a scary subject, but each day during your detox, you've got to meditate. Meditation is a time to simply sit still, with your body, breath, and thoughts. It doesn't have to be a scary thing or an extremely religious thing or some kind of out-of-body experience. In fact, I encourage you to make your meditations very much about your body. This is your chance to connect back with yourself and see where you might be holding tension, where your thoughts are leading you, and if your breath feels short. These simple things are your clues to some deeper things that might be going on within your own health and happiness.

Each day, morning and night, take five minutes to sit quietly. Close your eyes and sit still. Simply start to observe how you feel physically, emotionally, and mentally. For ten breaths, focus on your inhale and exhale. Feel each inhale and exhale growing steadier and deeper with each breath. Imagine each breath fills and then empties the lungs. After your ten breaths, come back to sitting still and find a bit of clarity in your thoughts. Repeat your daily intention, mantra, or phrase to yourself to keep your focus or to set your mindset for the day. You can also focus on a particular image in your mind that is meaningful to you.

That's it. When you connect your breath and allow your body to grow still, you start to notice negative thought patterns, cravings, or sensations within the body. Once you notice these things, you can focus on them and take the steps to remove anything that doesn't lead you to a happier, healthier place. Set a timer so you know when your few minutes are over, and if you feel the need, extend your time little by little each day. The more in tune you become with yourself, the easier it will be to notice the changes you are making and realize how health and happiness really feel.

After your meditation practice, take a few minutes to write down any thoughts, images, or emotions that came about during your meditation practice. If there was a recurring thought you had that day or an image that you kept seeing, write it down. If you felt distracted or your body felt tense, write it down. If you were feeling great and completely zen throughout your body, mind, and soul, write that down as well. It's OK to write down anything at all, whether you feel it is positive or negative—no one else is going to read this journal except for you. Sometimes simply getting things down on paper will help you to release the tension around the thought, image, or feeling and give you space to find more clarity in your life.

GROCERY LIST

No matter what your current diet or philosophy is (unless you are allergic to a specific food) throughout the next twenty-one days, there will be certain foods that you should avoid and certain foods that will be encouraged. These are the foods that either contribute to or rebuild a toxic system. You'll be taking a break from certain heavy, hard-to-digest, acidic foods. These include any animal product (including dairy, eggs, and meat), sugar, alcohol, most soy, wheat and gluten, and caffeine. All of these foods are acidic (even dairy) when they are consumed. This causes inflammation in the body, one of the main culprits to most major diseases, including heart disease, stroke, and cancer. They are all also hard to digest and can trigger gas, bloating, diarrhea, or constipation. Many times, people don't even realize they are having difficulty digesting these items until they are removed from their diet and they notice how much lighter and energetic they feel. Remember this: The foods to avoid are allergen triggers, digestive upsetters, and toxic overloaders. The foods to enjoy are foods that will be the basis of many of your recipes, since they are full of nutrients, vitamins, and energy.

Instead of focusing solely on what you can't buy, focus on what you can buy. You'll want to buy vegetables, especially leafy greens like kale and spinach; fruits such as berries, apples, and lemons; wheat- and gluten-free grains; beans and legumes; nuts and seeds. You'll also want to stock up on unsweetened nut milk (almond or coconut work well). You may also wish to purchase tempeh and tofu, soy products that are a little less processed and are high in protein. Tempeh is fermented, so it is easier to digest than tofu. Avoid "wheat meat," called seitan, as this is straight gluten and very hard to digest. Superfoods and spices are a great item to add to your shopping list, especially to support your system during your detox. These items include ground flax seeds, chia seeds, spirulina, hemp seeds as well as the spices turmeric, ginger, cinnamon, cardamom, and nutmeg. These are not necessary for the cleanse, but they do add *huge* amounts of nutritional value to some of the recipes.

Some of these are foods that might be new to you, so be open-minded and have fun with your new food experiments. And remember, you won't be avoiding all of these foods forever, this is just a way to reboot your system for the next three weeks so you will notice which of these foods you really do enjoy and how much you actually want them again after the cleanse. Use this list and the weekly meal plans to help you make your shopping lists for the next few weeks. Here is a sample grocery list of "do's" and "don'ts" on your cleanse:

Do's	Don'ts
Leafy greens	Wheat and gluten
Veggies	Meat
Fruits	Dairy
Juices (fresh)	Eggs
Smoothies (fresh, whole fruits and veggies)	Caffeine
	Sugar (processed or baked goods)
Quinoa and other gluten-free grains	Alcohol
Nuts and seeds	Limit soy to tofu, tempeh, or edamame 1–2 times per week
Beans and legumes (tofu, tempeh, and edamame are OK 1–2 times per week)	
	Store-bought, pasteurized juices and smoothies
Soups	
Salads	Canned soups

FOODS YOU SHOULD KNOW:

There are a few foods on your lists and recipes that you may not recognize. Here is a brief rundown on them.

Raw Agave Nectar: Agave nectar is a sweet substance that comes from the agave plant. When raw, it is a naturally, low-glycemic sweetener, which means that it sweetens without spiking your blood sugar.

Tofu: Tofu is a protein-based substance made from soybean curd. When organic, it is free of pesticides and is a fantastic source of protein and iron, especially if you are used to eating meat regularly. You can find it in the produce section of most grocery stores.

Tempeh: Tempeh is another soy-based product. It is made of fermented soybeans and sometimes mixed with brown rice or other grains. It comes as a solid block and is great for slicing into cubes or strips for recipes. It can be found with the tofu in most stores. (Make sure it is gluten-free, as some brands add barley and rice to the soybeans.)

Tamari: Tamari is a gluten-free soy sauce. Most traditional soy sauces also contain wheat, which is not gluten-free.

Nutritional Yeast: Also known as "cheezy flakes," nutritional yeast can be found at most health foods stores and often in the bulk bin section at these stores. It is a flaky substance that can be sprinkled onto your dishes or made into a sauce for cheese-type sauces and dips.

Kale: Kale is the king of the leafy greens. It packs more nutrition per bite than any other food around. You'll use kale in many of your recipes, including your juices and smoothies. You can find it in your produce section with the lettuces and other greens, such as collards.

Quinoa: Quinoa is a grain-like seed that can be used in any dish that would normally call for rice. It is a complete protein, which is rare for most plants. This means that it is high in protein and contains all the essential amino acid building blocks your system needs.

Tahini: Tahini is sesame seed paste. It can be used in many recipes, like any nut or seed butter, but in this program it is mostly used in your salad dressings.

Chia and Flax Seeds: Chia and flax seeds are tiny seeds that are full of healthy fats. They can be used in baked goods or in certain recipes as a binder, because they become gelatinous when soaked in liquid.

Chlorophyll: Chlorophyll is abundant in all green vegetables and is what allows the plants to feed and grow from the sun. It packs your green vegetables full of vitamins and nutrients, making them superfoods and energy-builders.

Spirulina: Spirulina is a blue-green algae that is high in protein and B vitamins. Spirulina can be found in a powdered form, which can be added to smoothies, protein bars, and other recipes.

SPICES YOU'LL LOVE

DIGESTION

Some spices can be used to increase digestion and ease any indigestion you may be experiencing. Cinnamon is one of these common spices and can be used in drinks and remedies. Ginger is another of these spices and it is commonly used, along with cinnamon, as a flavor-enhancer but also as a digestive aide. These can be used in herbal teas or in foods, smoothies, and juices to help increase your digestion.

MELLOW OUT

Some spices can be used to help you relax and stay calm during moments of stress or an accidental caffeine overload. Nutmeg and cardamom are both spices that can be used to help calm and relax you, leading to better sleep or just a less jittery state of mind. Before the cleanse, you can add these to your coffee to help decrease any jitters or caffeine crashes and to help wean you off coffee. They can also be used in a mug of warmed coconut or almond milk in the evening to help you settle in before bed.

INFLAMMATION REDUCER

Turmeric is a great spice that can be used to reduce inflammation. It can be added to a variety of dishes and is used in a few of the recipes in this book.

Chapter Three: Preparing for Your Detox

Before you begin your program, you'll want to take some time to prepare yourself physically and mentally for the changes and challenges you are about to undergo. Although this plan will guide you step by step, there will still be times when you might feel like you want give up completely or rush ahead to get it over with. In order to prevent this, prepare yourself *before* you start the process with a few simple steps and tweaks. If you dive head first into your detox, you could wind up with variety of negative physical and mental issues, including headaches, bellyaches, fatigue, mental stress, and an overall frantic feeling. Not exactly what you are looking for during your restorative program, right?

A week before you want to begin the program, start to prepare. Follow the recipes and/or meal plans to make a grocery list. Figure out what foods you will need and where the best place to buy them is. Health foods stores are your best bet, but you may need to find out where the closest one is. Farmers markets are also a fantastic and economical way to get plenty of fresh, and often organic, fruits and veggies. Map out the days you can go to the grocery store and when the

farmers markets are open in your area. Make a plan about how many times a week you will need to head to the store and where you can fit it into your schedule. You might want or need to make one big trip, or you may stop by the store several times a week as needed.

In the week(s) before your cleanse, start to physically prepare for the cleanse by eliminating trigger foods. Slowly start to take away some of the foods you know are "banned" for the next few weeks and add in some of the "super power" foods you'll be eating more of. These are the foods located in the *Do's and Don'ts* chart on page 7. This will help your body prepare for the changes in your diet, and it will also give you time to figure out which flavors and recipes you like the best.

Allow yourself plenty of time to start removing them from your diet as you add in more fresh produce. Slowly wean off dairy, processed or packaged foods, wheat and gluten (even bread), and meat. Take your time in doing this, so it doesn't feel as if you are depriving yourself or restricting your intake. Slowly eliminate one thing at a time from your diet. Begin to eliminate dairy and meat from your diet first. These are often the staples of our American diet and are the biggest emotional triggers when we try to let go of them. If you eat meat at most meals and have a glass of milk along with it, see if you can slowly switch to something else to prepare for the week. Try water or unsweetened tea for your drinks. Add in larger portions of vegetables to help decrease the amount of meat you are eating. Use green or black tea to help you kick the caffeine habit. And try to reduce the amount of alcohol you consume, especially if you consume it daily. Sugar is the really tricky one. Sugar acts like a drug in our system. When we eat it, it hooks us in and we crave more. It makes us feel great and energized, and then we crash and crave more and the cycle continues. Slowly switch sugary snacks and drinks out for fresh fruits and juices. Use agave, maple syrup, or even honey instead of white table sugar.

All of these tiny changes will help to minimize the mental fatigue and physical discomfort that can go along with the beginnings of a detox. While you are removing a few things from your eating plan, start to add in more fresh fruits and vegetables and shift your focus to the additions to your diet, rather than the things you are removing. This will help you to focus on all the good things you can eat, while you crowd out the things that won't be available for the twenty-one-day program. The more you enjoy the healthy foods you are adding in, the more likely you are to keep eating them. It's as simple as that. If you start to do this

ahead of time, you'll not only be prepared when the cleanse comes around, but you'll also already be on your way to making lasting habits and changes for life.

Set aside time to prepare for your detox. Start to carve out time in your schedule to prepare your meals and snacks, exercise, and meditate. If you start before the cleanse actually begins, you'll have more time to dedicate to your health, rather than creating stress. Make sure you have about five minutes at the beginning and end of each day, an hour or so to move your body, and enough time to prepare whatever healthy dishes you decide to eat that day. Leftovers can come in handy before or after the cleanse on occasion, but during it you want your foods as fresh as possible so the digestive enzymes can help support you and detox your system.

It's also a good idea to start to prepare your loved ones. They may not realize what a detox is and they may assume that you can't eat *anything* or they might assume that you are still eating *everything*. If you explain and prepare ahead of time, they'll be more likely to support you or even join you in some of the process. Prepare them for the change in not only your food choices but also in the lifestyle habits you are creating. You might not be available to stay up late watching TV or you might not sleep in quite as late in the mornings. Simply explain to them the reasons behind your choices and give them a peek at the book. Let them know that you might not be able to grab a glass of wine or a cup of coffee with them over the next few weeks, but you'd love to join them for a cup of tea. If you are the main chef for your household, let your family know that some of the meals they are eating may have more vegetables, or that they may need to help cook some other foods. And most importantly, let them all know that you are doing this to become a happier, healthier you, which means that you are going to need them to lean on for support and lots of love through this process. You might even invite them to join you on your journey!

Chapter Four:
Exercise Plans and Programs

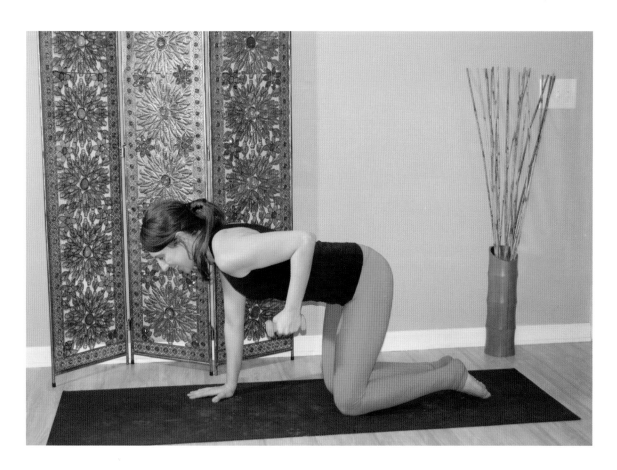

During the next twenty-one days, you'll be exercising to help release toxins, move them out of your body, and reenergize your system. The first week will be gentle in order to ease you into exercising this way and support your system through the more intense detoxification week. In the second week, you'll exercise at a more intense pace, but still more gentle than you might be used to, to build energy and detoxify your system further. In the third week, you'll slow down your pace slightly to help you stay energized as you incorporate all of your food and workouts into your post-detox plan.

Exercise Plan	Monday	Tuesday	Wednesday	Thursday	Friday	Saturday	Sunday
Week 1	Detox Yoga	Stretchy Yoga	Stretchy Yoga	Detox Yoga	Stretchy Yoga	Detox Yoga	Stretchy Yoga
Week 2	Energy Sculpt	Detox Yoga	Stretchy Yoga	Energy Sculpt	Detox Yoga	Energy Sculpt (or favorite workout)	Detox Yoga
Week 3	Detox Yoga	Stretchy Yoga	Energy Sculpt	Detox Yoga	Energy Sculpt	Stretchy Yoga	Detox Yoga

PROGRAMS

ENERGY SCULPT

You will need light 2–3 pound weights for this exercise. If you do not have weights, you can always use water bottles or perform the exercise without weights.

Warm-Up

Seated Breath and Twists
Come to a comfortable cross-legged position, sitting on your mat. Lengthen your spine to sit tall with the chest open. Inhale as you reach your arms out and overhead. Exhale as you reach them back down. Repeat this five times.

Inhale your arms back over head, but this time, as you exhale, twist to the right, bringing your left hand to your right knee and your right hand behind your

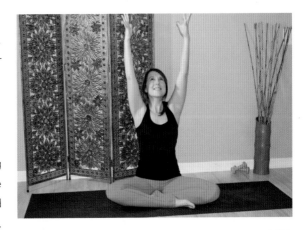

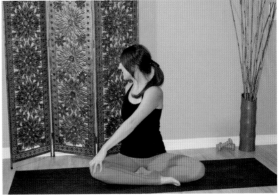

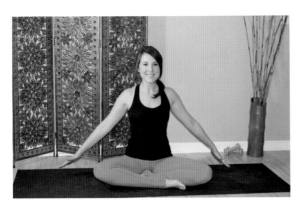

spine. Inhale to reach your arms back up to the center and, as you exhale, twist to the left. The right hand comes across your knee and the left hand reaches behind you. Repeat this for five rounds.

Cat/Cow

After your last exhale, come onto your hands and knees. Bring your knees six inches apart under your hips and bring your wrists directly under your shoulders. As you inhale, lift your chest and hips up while you release your belly. On your exhale, push your hand into the mat and pull your belly button into your spine as you round your back. Repeat five times.

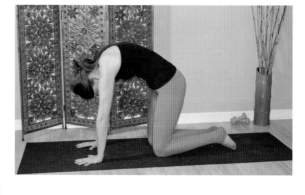

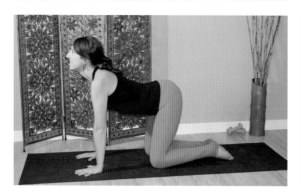

Leg and Arm Balance

Come back to hands and knees. Find a neutral spine by pulling your belly button toward your spine. Reach your right leg straight back from the hip and your left arm forward. Pull the belly up and in a little more for support. Hold for five breaths and release. Switch sides and repeat.

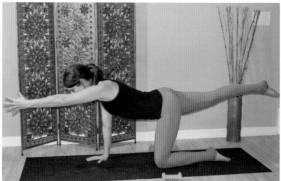

Plank and Downward-Facing Dog

From hands and knees, step your feet back and lift your knees to come in to plank pose (a.k.a. the top of a push-up). Squeeze your thighs, push through your heels, and engage the lower abdominals by pulling them up and in. Take an inhale. As you exhale press into your hands and push your hips up toward the ceiling into downward-facing dog. Inhale back to plank. Exhale to downward dog. Repeat this five times.

Walk Back with Squat

From downward-facing dog, walk your hands back to meet your feet. Squat down and lift your heels, Keep your knees together. Grab your weights and bring your hands down on either side of your feet. Slowly push into your heels and roll all the way up to standing.

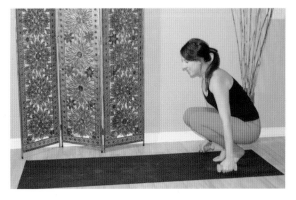

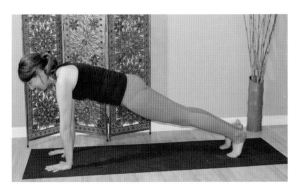

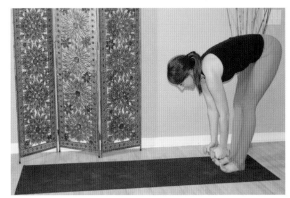

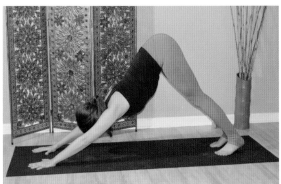

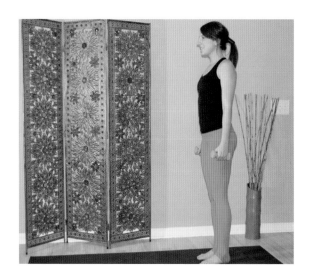

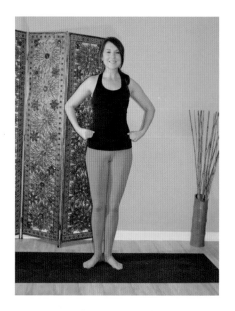

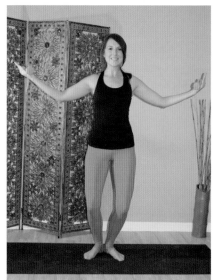

Standing Series

Small Plié with Reach Up and Down, Bicep Half Curls

Bring your heels together with your toes turned open. Draw your navel toward your spine to help lengthen your lower back and support your spine. Turn your palms and weights to face up. Bend your knees and reach your arms to the height of your shoulders. Turn your palms to face down as your press your hands back to your sides and lengthen your legs. Repeat this twelve times.

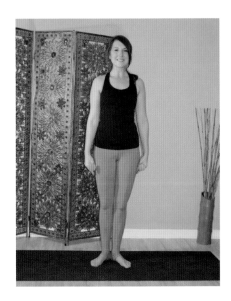

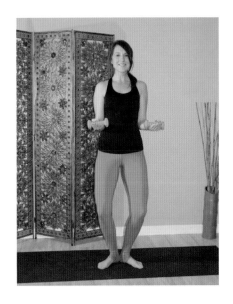

Bend your knees and hold them bent. Keep your navel drawing toward your spine. Lift your arms to a ninety-degree angle with your palms facing up. Hug your elbows and upper arms into your sides. Keep your knees bent as you slowly bend your elbows, bringing the weights to your shoulders. Release back down to ninety degrees. Repeat twelve times. After the twelfth time, hold the arm bend for eight counts.

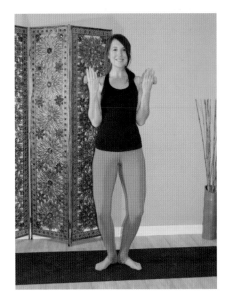

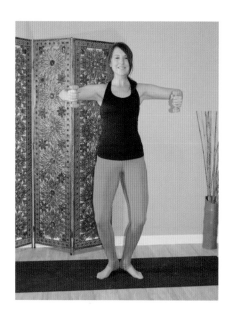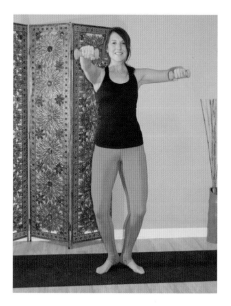

Slowly lift your heels until they just hover above the ground. You'll really want to firm up the core, pelvis, and inner thighs for this exercise. Keeping your arms at ninety-degree angles, lift your elbows out to the height of your shoulders. As you lift up, the palm will start to face in. Then hug your elbows back into your sides to lower. As you hug them back in, feel the sides of your torso squeezing to hug them back into place. Repeat twelve times and hold on the last round with the elbows lifted.

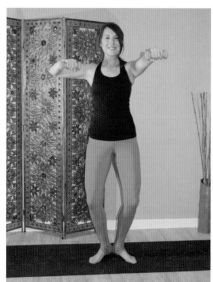

Turn your weights to face down by rotating your wrists slightly. Keep your heels lifted, your core engaged, and your spine long. Reach your arms forward, straightening the arms and bringing your weights together. Slowly pull back to start. Repeat twelve times. After the twelfth time, alternate your reach side to side, reaching to just the right, then just the left. You can add a little twist of your torso as you reach, but keep your hip and legs still.

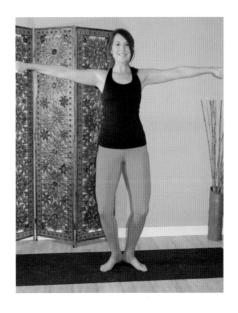

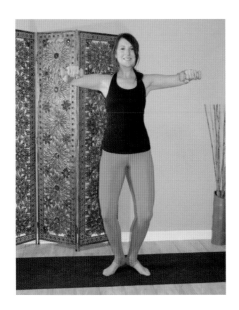

Pull both elbows back and lower your heels. Slowly lengthen your arms out to the side and then bend your elbows again. Repeat this twelve times. And release your arms down.

Wide Plié Arm Circles and Pulses

Step open to a wide plié stance, with your heels two to three feet apart and knees wider than your hips. Bend your knees until your thighs are almost parallel to the ground and your knees come over your ankles. Make sure to keep your belly button pulling in toward the spine, your lower back lengthened, and your heart lifted. Reach your weights behind you with your palms facing in toward your glutes. Push into your heels to straighten your legs and reach your arms out and up over head. Bend your knees as you press your arms back behind you. Repeat this for eight rounds. Hold at the bottom of the move.

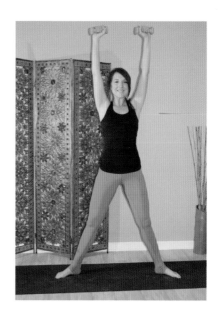

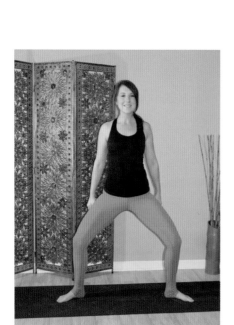

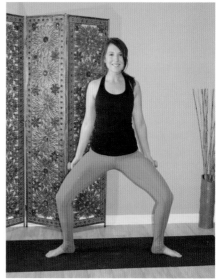

Pulse your weights together for twelve counts. Turn your palms to face each other and pulse your weights back for twelve counts.

Squat V's with Pulse and Lift

Reach your arms back as high as you can and hinge at your hips as you lean forward to a flat back. You'll want to keep your heart reaching forward and up slightly and your core engaged for support. Slowly reach your arms forward and up as you lengthen your legs and stand tall. Bend your knees, hinge at your hips, and reach your arms back behind you again. Repeat eight times.

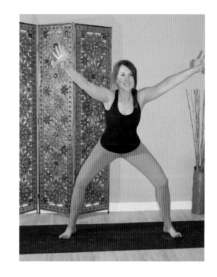

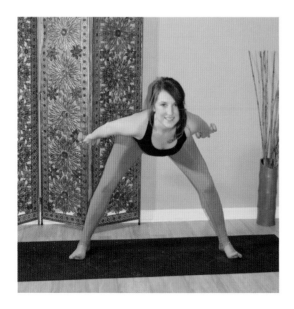

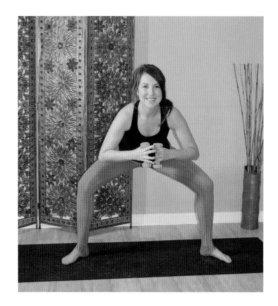

After the eighth time, hold the squat and bring the weights together at your chest in Namaste hands. Slightly lower your hips and pulse for twelve counts. After the last pulse, hold.

Push into your heels to straighten your legs. Lift your heart and reach your arms straight out. Push back down into your squat. Repeat this twelve times.

Chair Pose with Shoulder/Tricep Bend and Extension
Step your feet together and sit into a squat. Keep your navel drawing up and in toward your spine for support and your collar bone broad to release tension in the neck and shoulders. Pulse here for twelve counts.

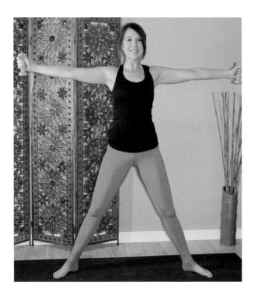

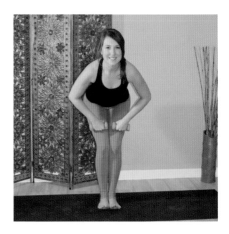

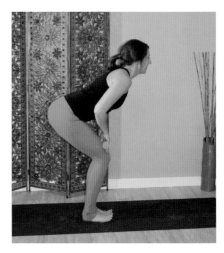

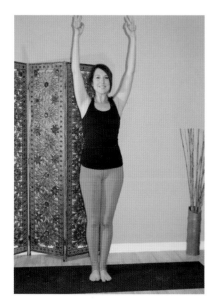

Slowly reach your arms straight up by your ears as you stand tall. Lower back into your squat and reach your arms behind you. Lift straight back up and lower again. Repeat twelve times total. On the last round, hold in the squat with your arms reaching back.

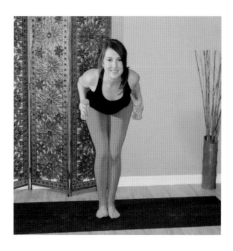

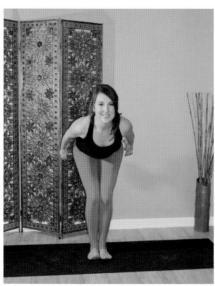

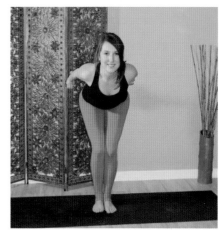

Lift your chest slightly and drop your hips a little lower. Keep your upper arms still and bend your elbows. Lengthen back out. Repeat twelve times.

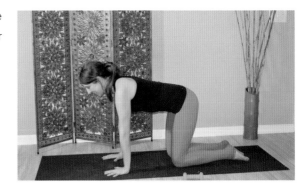

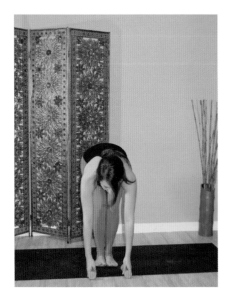

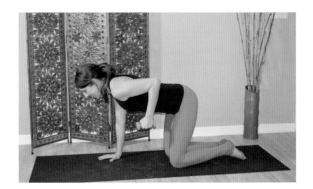

Slowly squat all the way to the ground and release your weights. Come back to hands and knees on our mat.

Floor Series
Hands and Knees with Tricep Bend and Extension
On your hands and knees, grab onto your weight with your right hand. Bend your right elbow and hug your upper arm into your side. Extend your arm straight. Keep the upper arm still as you re-bend your elbow. Repeat twelve times and lower your weight.

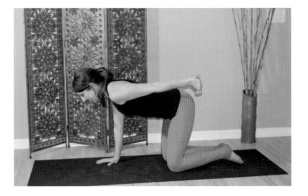

Diagonal Reach, Leg Pulse, and Arm Circles

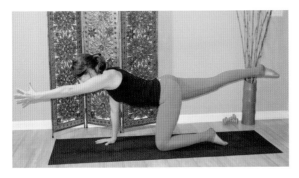

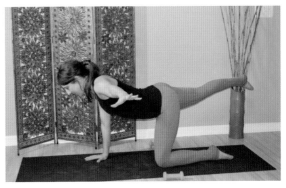

Slowly reach your arm straight out to the side, keep your leg lifted, and make tiny circles forward with the arm. Make eight circles and reverse your direction for another eight counts.

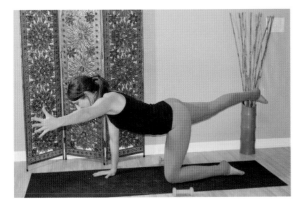

Reach your arm straight ahead and lift your left leg off the ground. Draw your navel into your spine to support the lower back. Inhale as you reach our arm and leg out to the corners of your mat. Exhale as your reach back to the start. Repeat twelve times.

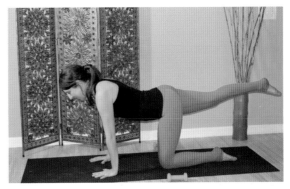

Bring your hand down to the ground and pulse your leg up and down for a count of twelve.

Side-to-Side Hip Lift

Keep both hands on the ground. Turn your left hip open and draw your knee in toward your elbow. Lengthen back out. Repeat eight times.

Repeat the previous three exercises on the other side.

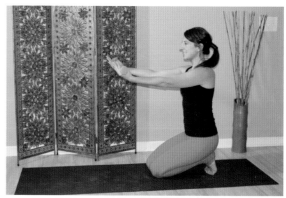

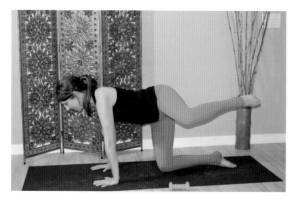

Kneeling Arm Reach

Come to a kneeling position with your weights in your hands. Sweep your arms up to the height of your shoulders with your palms facing up. Slowly pull your arms back down, hugging your elbows back. Repeat this twelve times, keeping your elbows slightly bent and your core engaged throughout.

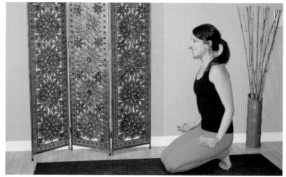

Lean Back with Alternate Arm Extension

Come to stand on your knees. If needed, roll up your mat under your knees for cushioning.

With the weights in your hands, reach your arms straight ahead at the height of your shoulders. Keep your core strong and lean back, hinging at your knees. As you lean back, open your left arm out to the side.

Squeeze through your core to lift back up and bring your arm back forward. Repeat five times and switch arms. Release your weights and take a seat.

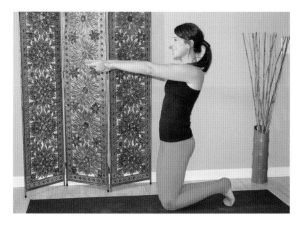

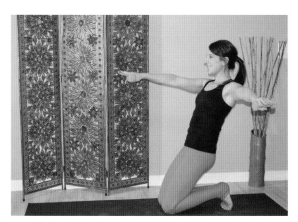

Boat Scoops

Sit with your knees bent and the soles of your feet on the ground. Bring your knees together. As you breathe in, reach your arms up and lengthen your spine. As you breathe out, pull your elbows into your sides and scoop your belly. Inhale to lift, exhale to scoop. Repeat twelve times. On your last round, hold the scoop.

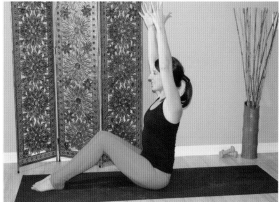

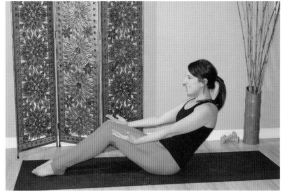

Wave Watcher

Lower your elbows down to the ground next to your hips. Keep your core scooped and contracted. Make sure you don't sink into your shoulders here by lifting the chest slightly. Extend your right leg to hover an inch off the ground. Lift your right leg up and then lower. Pull your knee toward your chest and extend. Repeat eight times, lifting up, lowering, knee in, and back out. Switch sides and repeat.

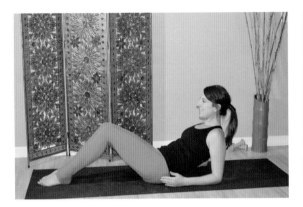
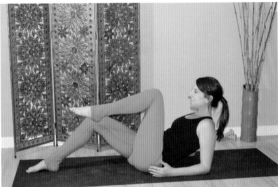

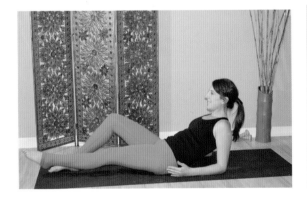
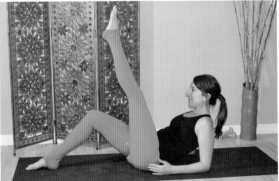

Bridge with Leg Lifts

Roll down to the mat. Walk your heels in under your knees. Keep your knees and feet hips distance apart. Place your hands by your hips. Slowly scoop up your spine and lift your hips toward the ceiling into bridge pose. Hold your hips high and reach your right leg up toward the ceiling. Engage your core to help hold you steady. Keep your right leg long as you press it down toward the ground and back up. Repeat five times and switch sides. After your last round, roll all the way down to the ground and turn onto your stomach.

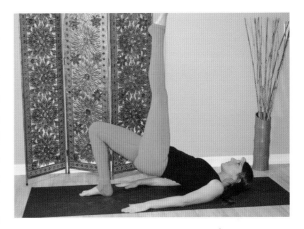

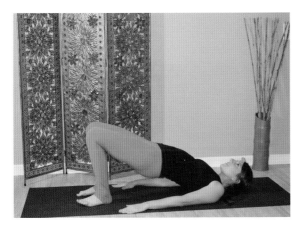

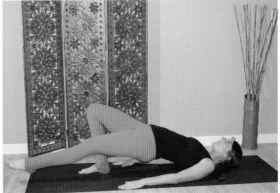

Forearm Plank

Place your elbows under your shoulders with your arms parallel. Tuck your toes, lift your knees, and come off the ground into a forearm plank pose. Draw your belly button up and in as you slightly draw your bottom ribs toward your hip bones. Hold for five breaths and release down.

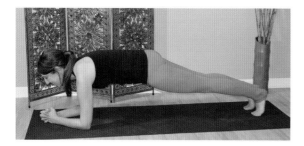

Sphinx Roll Up

Stay on your forearms with your heart lifted. Squeeze your legs together. Slowly draw your belly button into your spine, lift your pelvis off the mat, and lift your hip flexors and the tops of the thighs. Your knees will stay on the ground here. Hold for five counts and lower back down. Repeat five times.

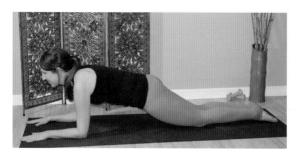

Cool Down

Sphinx

Separate your legs out to the corners of your mat. With your forearms on the mat, lift your heart forward and up to stretch the front of your core. Hold for three breaths and lower down to the mat.

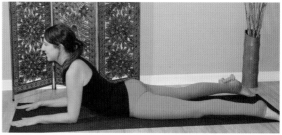

Downward-Facing Dog with Alternating Heels

Tuck your toes, push into your hands, and lift your hips up and back to downward-facing dog. Hold for three breaths. Slightly bend your left knee and press your right heel toward the ground to deepen the stretch up the back of your leg. Hold for two breaths and switch sides.

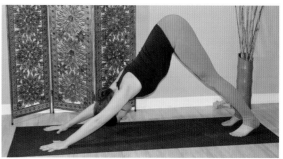

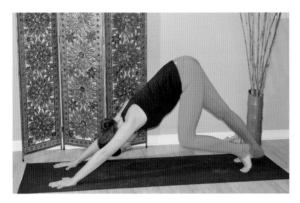

Wide Child's Pose
Bring your knees down to the edges of the mat with your big toes touching. Sit your hips onto your heels and fold forward onto the mat. Hold for five breaths.

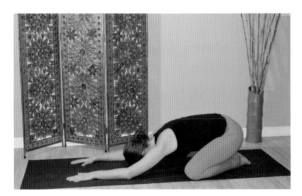

Kneeling Arm Stretches: Shoulders, Triceps, and Biceps
Come to a kneeling position, with the knees together and the hips on the heels. Reach your right arm down to the ground and the left arm up toward the ceiling.

Lean over to the right and let your left arm reach up and overhead as you lean. Hold for three breaths and switch sides.

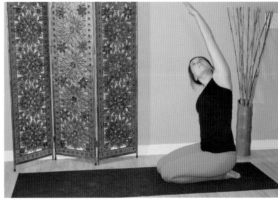

Clasp your hands in front of you and press your palms away as you round your back. Hold for three breaths and release.

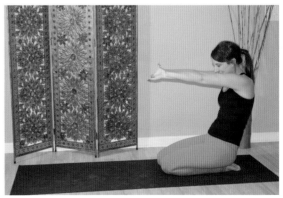

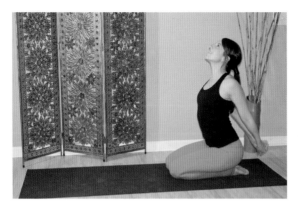

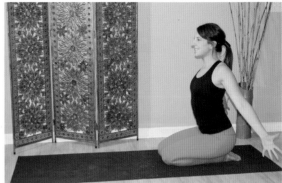

Clasp your hands behind you with the palms facing each other. Lift your arms away from you and let your shoulders roll back. Hold for three breaths and release.

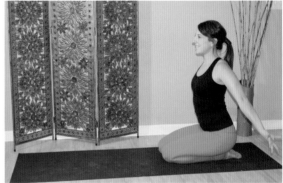

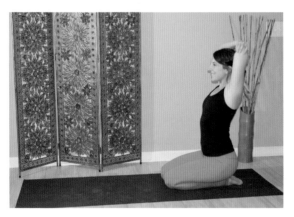

Reach your right arm up toward the ceiling. Bend your elbow and reach your finger tips down between your shoulder blades. Press your elbow back further with your left hand. Hold for three breaths and switch sides.

Stretch your arms out to the sides and rotate them five times.

Forward Fold

Bring your legs forward and sit with a tall spine. If needed, you can sit on a blanket or pillow or roll up your mat to lengthen even more. Hinge from your hips and fold over your legs. Keep your spine long by reaching your chest toward your shins and your gaze toward your ankles. Your hands can reach for your toes or shins. Hold for five breaths.

Half Forward Fold and Reach Back

Lift out of your forward fold and bring your right leg over to the right edge of your mat. Turn over your leg and fold with a long spine, just as you did in the previous fold. Hold for three breaths. After the third breath, reach your left arm up and behind you. Push into your right foot, lift your hips, and stretch your right arm behind you. Hold for one breath and lower. Repeat both stretches on the opposite side.

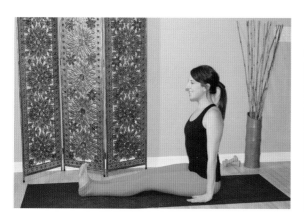

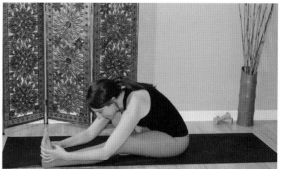

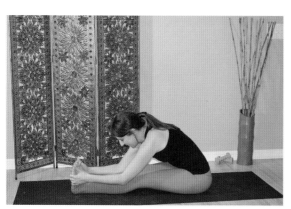

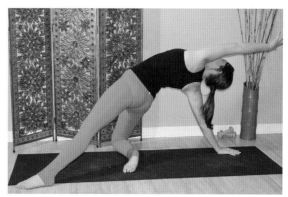

Cobblers Pose

Bring the soles of your feet together and clasp your hands around your feet. Lift your chest and start to lean forward. Hold for three breaths and release.

Seated Breaths

Come back to a cross-legged position and lengthen your spine. On an inhale reach your arms overhead. As you exhale, press them back down. Take another breath in as your reach up and exhale back down. On the last round, inhale and reach up, bringing your palms together. Exhale and bring your hands to your heart to finish your workout.

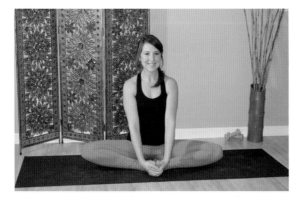

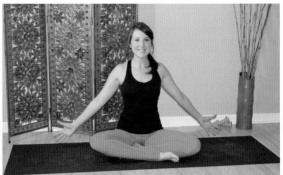

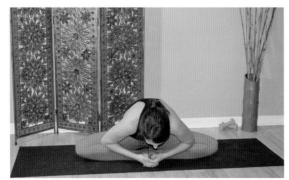

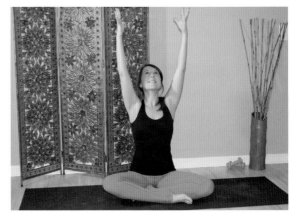

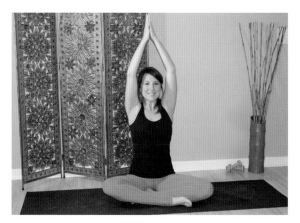

DETOX YOGA

Warm-Up

Knees to Chest

Lie on your back with our knees drawn into your chest. Wrap your arms around your knees and grab opposite elbows, forearms, or wrists. Try to keep your lower back and head on the ground as you do this. Make small circles in each direction, three to each side.

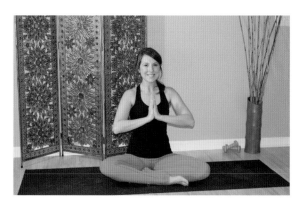

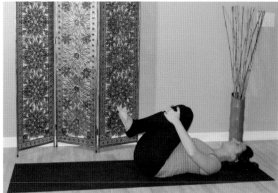

Side to Side Twists with Breath

Release your hands and bring your arms out to a "T" shape. Bring your knees over your hips. Inhale as you lower your knees down to the right, hovering above the ground. Exhale as you lift back to center. Inhale as you drop your knees to the left, hovering about the ground. Exhale back to center. Repeat five times on each side.

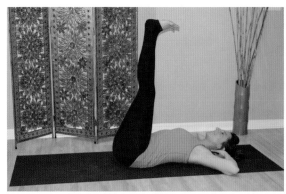

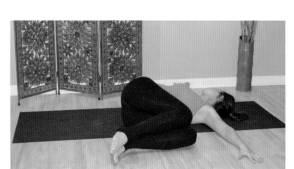

Crunching Leg Lift

From the center, reach your legs up toward the ceiling and flex your feet. Bring your hands behind your head with your elbows wide. Inhale flat onto the mat and exhale to peel your head and shoulders off the mat. Inhale to lower back down. Repeat ten times. Draw your knees into your chest.

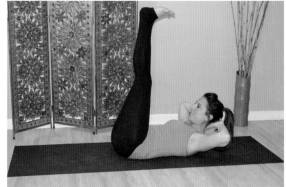

One-Legged Lift and Twist

Reach your left leg down onto the mat and flex your foot. Hug your right knee into your chest as you clasp your hands around your shin. Inhale and lengthen your spine onto the mat. Exhale and push your shin into your hands, draw your knee over your hip, and lift your head and shoulders off the mat. Inhale to lower, and exhale to lift. Repeat for five rounds. After the fifth round, lower your head and twist your right knee across your body to the left. Reach your right arm out to the side and turn your head to the right. Hold for five breaths. Draw both knees back into the center and repeat on the left side.

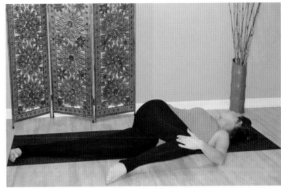

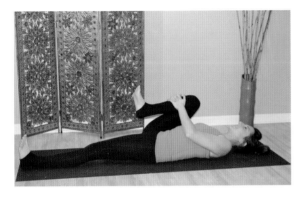

Roll Up

Hug both knees into your chest and draw your forehead into your knees. Draw your belly button into your spine and rock front to back until you come up to seated.

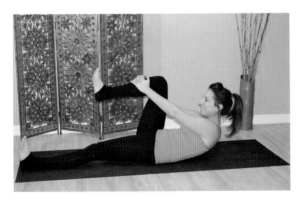

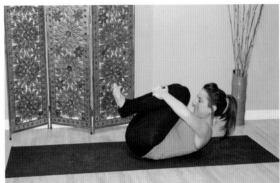

Seated Breath with Twists

Sit in a cross-legged position. Inhale as you reach your arms overhead. Exhale and twist to the right, bringing your right arm behind you and your left arm to the outer edge of your right leg. Lengthen your spine. Inhale reach back up. Exhale to twist to the left. Repeat five times.

Cat/Cow

After your last round, come onto hands and knees. Bring your wrists under your shoulders and your knees under your hips. Inhale as you lift your heart and your hips. Exhale as you round your back, drawing your navel to your spine. Repeat five times.

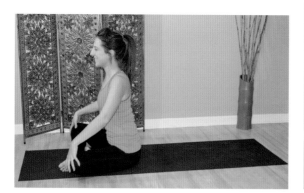

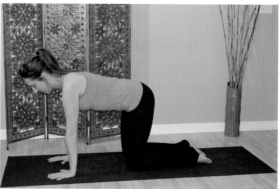

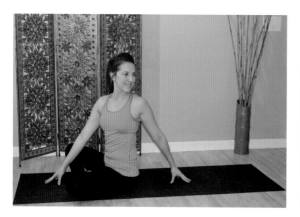

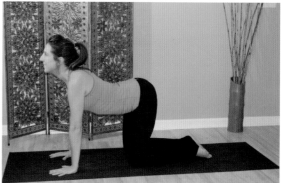

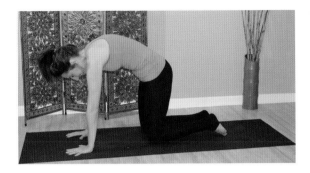

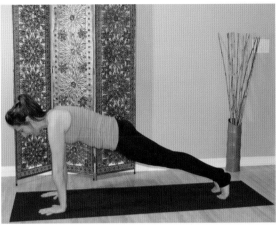

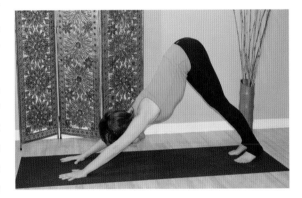

Downward-Facing Dog to Plank

After the fifth round, step your right foot straight back, then the left, to come into plank pose. Keep your shoulders in line over your wrists. Squeeze your quadriceps to lengthen your knees and press through your heels. Draw your navel up and in toward your spine. Hold for three breaths.

Exhale and press back to downward-facing dog. Keep your hands and feet where they are. Press your hips toward the ceiling, while drawing your chest toward your thighs and your heels down toward the ground. Keep your fingers spread wide and push your hands into the mat. Keep squeezing your thighs to push your heels down. Hold for five breaths. After five breaths, inhale forward to plank. Exhale back to downward dog. Repeat ten times. After the tenth time, hold for three more breaths in downward dog.

Rag Doll

Walk your feet toward your hands and fold over your legs. Relax your arms toward the ground or grab opposite elbows. Relax your head and neck. Hold for ten breaths. After the last round of breath, slowly release your hands and roll up to standing. Let your head be the last thing to lift up.

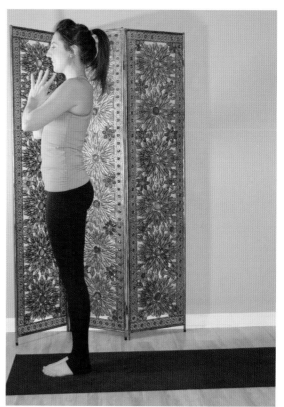

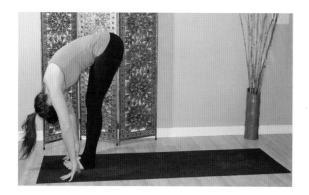

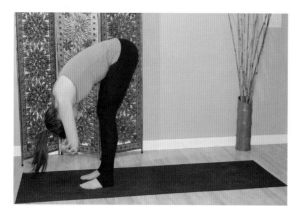

Sun Salutations

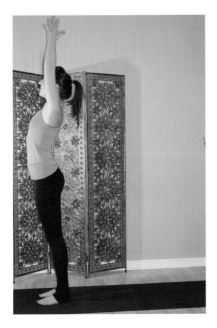

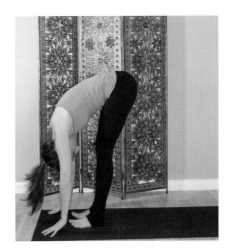

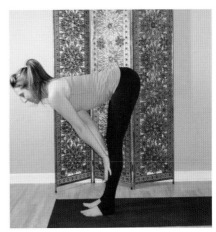

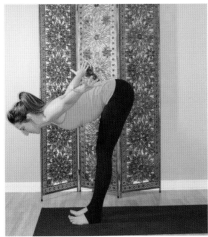

Inhale as you reach your arms overhead. Exhale as you dive forward into a fold. Inhale to bring your hands to your shins and lengthen your spine in a halfway lift. Exhale and fold. Inhale and reach your arms out and up to stand. Repeat three times total.

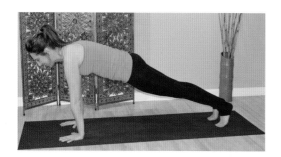

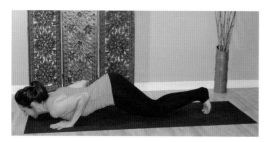

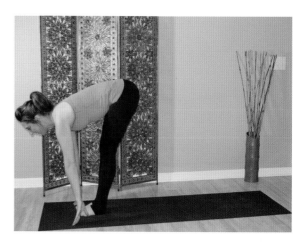

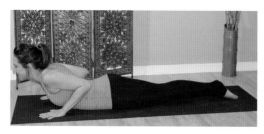

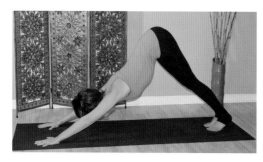

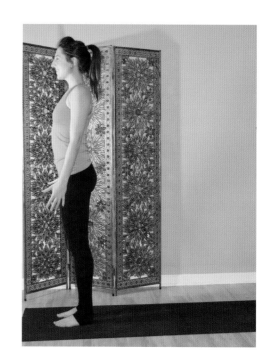

After the third time, dive forward into your fold. Inhale hands to your shins. Exhale step back to a plank pose. Bring your wrists under your shoulders, press your heels back to lengthen your spine, and squeeze your legs. Draw your belly button into your spine. Take a breath in. As you exhale, lower your knees to the ground, hug your elbows and upper arms into your sides, and lower your torso evenly. Inhale to press your pelvis and belly into the mat as you lift your chest and rib cage into Baby Cobra. Exhale to tuck your toes, push into your hands, and send your hips back to downward dog. Hold for three breaths. On your next inhale, look forward and step to your hands. Exhale fold. Inhale reach up and out to stand.

Repeat this series three times total.

Chair Twist

Bring your palms together at your heart. Sink your hips back and down like you're sitting in a chair. Lean forward to almost a flat back. Keep your hips and legs steady as you twist to the right, bringing your left elbow and upper arm across your right thigh. Your palms will stay pressing together here. Hold for three breaths and release into a forward fold. Step your feet hips distance apart and wrap your arms behind your knees, grabbing your opposite elbows. Draw your head in close to your knees as you soften your belly. Hold for five breaths. Walk your feet back together, bend your knees, lift your torso and arms, sit back into chair pose. Repeat on the left side.

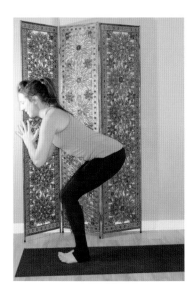
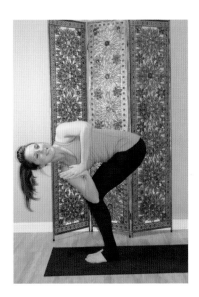
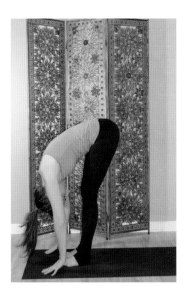

Chair Twist Power-Up

Inhale as you lengthen your legs and reach your hands overhead, with your palms together. Exhale into a chair twist to the right. Inhale to reach up. Exhale and twist to the left. Repeat this sequence ten times. After the final twist, forward fold to release your spine.

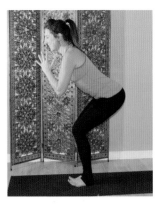

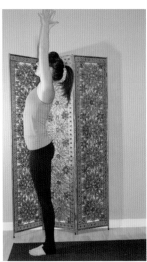

Warrior Series

Lunge to Twist

Bring your hands or fingertips to the mat and step your left foot back to a lunge. Keep your heel lifted off the ground and squeeze your left thigh for balance. Bring your right thigh parallel to the ground with your knee over your ankle. You may need to shift the left leg further back to do so. Draw your belly button into your spine and hug your inner thighs to the center for stability. Lift up and bring your hands to the center of your chest. Slowly lean forward and twist to the right, bringing your left arm across the right leg. Keep squeezing the inner thighs for balance. Hold for two breaths.

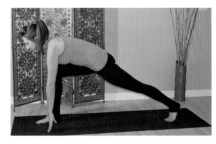

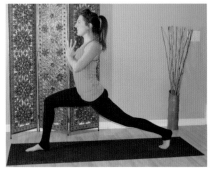

Warrior II

Slowly lift back to the center as you pivot your heel down to the ground. Reach your arms open to a "T" and turn your torso open to the left into warrior II. Hold for three breaths.

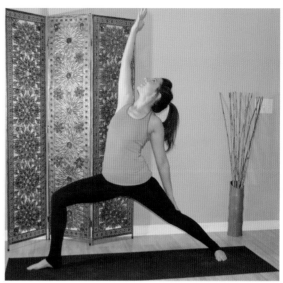

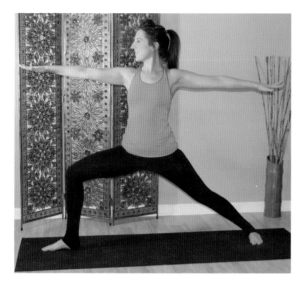

Alternating Reverse Warrior and Extended Side Angle
Flip your front palm so that it faces up. Inhale and reach your left arm to your back leg and your right arm up to the ceiling in reverse warrior. Hold for two breaths. Exhale and bring your right forearm to your right inner thigh into extended side angle. Reach your left arm straight up to the ceiling. Hold for two breaths. Inhale and reach back. Exhale reach forward. Repeat for five rounds. Come back to warrior II.

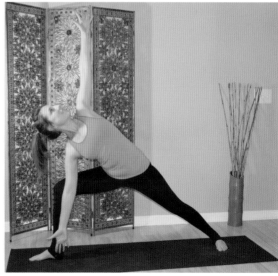

Triangle and Pyramid Pose Reach

Straighten your right leg. Press your right hip crease back and let your left hip lift up. Shift your ribcage to the right and reach your right fingertips forward. Rotate your right fingertips down to your shin and your left fingertips up to the ceiling into triangle. Hold for two breaths. Inhale in this pose and exhale as you reach your left hand toward your right big toe and rotate your chest toward the mat, moving into pyramid. Inhale to reach back open. Repeat five times. After the last round, plant your hands, bend your right knee, and step back to downward dog. Hold for three breaths. Step your left foot forward and repeat the sequence on the left side, ending in a fold.

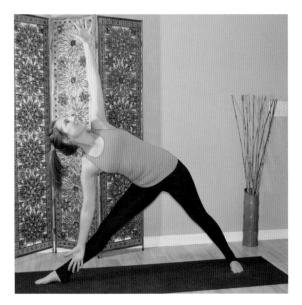
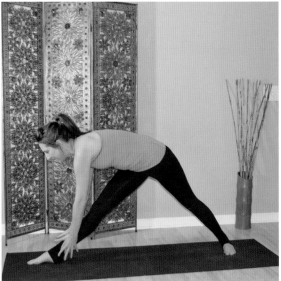

Wide-Legged Chair Series

Lift Up with Heel Lift to Skier
Step your feet hips distance apart. Bend your knees and lift to a wide-legged chair pose. Keep your knees over your ankles at hips distance. Reach your arms straight back behind you and come to a flat back. Lift your heels as you reach your arms overhead and lift to standing. Exhale and fold back into your wide-legged chair. Inhale and reach back up. Repeat five times. End in a forward fold.

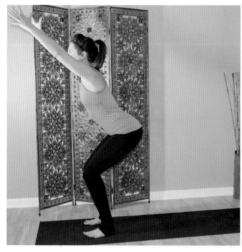

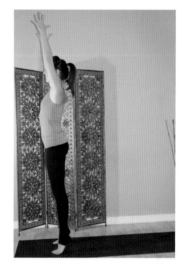

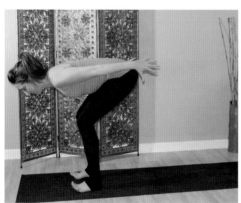

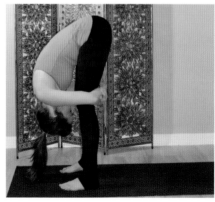

Lunge Series

Lunge to Hand Down Twist

Step your left foot back into a lunge. See previous lunge for details. Keep your hands on the ground. Spin your right arm up and open into a twist. Keep your left hand or fingertips on the ground. Hold for three breaths. Bring your hands down on either side of your front foot and lower your back knee to the mat.

Low Lunge to Half Hanumanasana

Keep your right knee over your ankle as you press your hips forward and down toward your right heel. Draw your navel into your spine and reach your arms up as you lift your torso into a low lunge. Hold for three breaths. Lower your hands back down and slide your hips back, stacking your right hip over your right knee. Your right leg will straighten. Flex your foot and fold forward over your leg. Hold for three breaths.

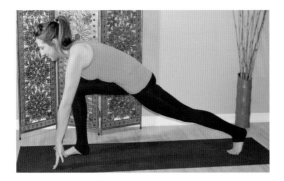

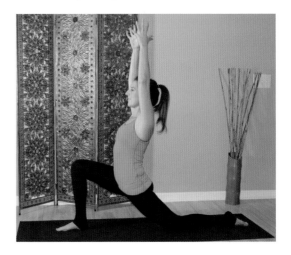

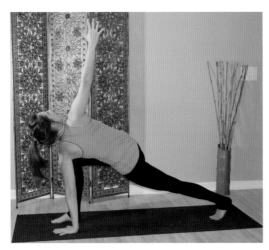

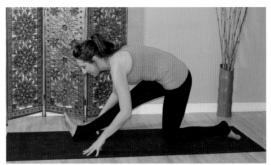

Lizard Pose

Slowly shift forward into your low lunge again. Bring both hands down to your mat next to the inside of your front foot. Shift your right foot over to the edge of your mat. Come down onto your forearms as you let your right knee turn out to the side. Hold here for five breaths.

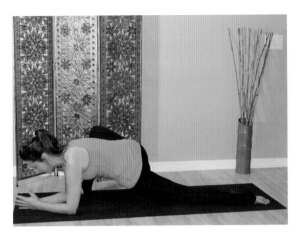

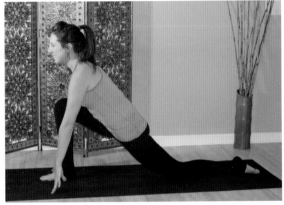

Wide Fold

Come back onto your hands, tuck your back toes, and lift your back knee. Pivot around to the left side of your mat and turn your toes into parallel. Lengthen your spine and fold forward. Hold for three breaths.

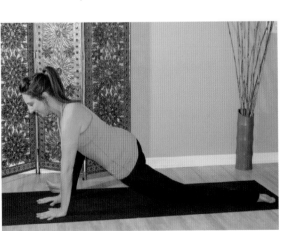

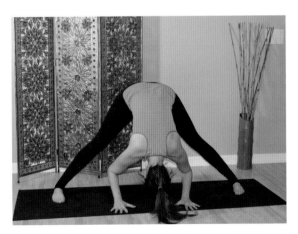

High Lunge to Warrior III

Shift back around to your lunge with your back heel off the mat. Lift your torso and reach your arms up overhead. Hold for three breaths. Draw your navel into your spine as you bring your hands to your heart. Slowly lean forward to a flat back. Keep pressing out through your heel and squeeze your left thigh. Shift your weight into your right foot as you lift you left leg off the mat. Come to hip height with your torso and your leg so you are parallel to the ground. Hold for three breaths.

Step your feet together and forward fold for five breaths. Repeat the entire sequence on the opposite side.

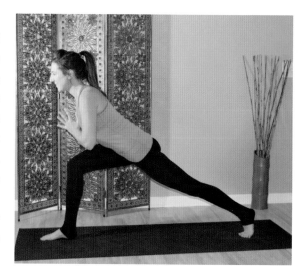

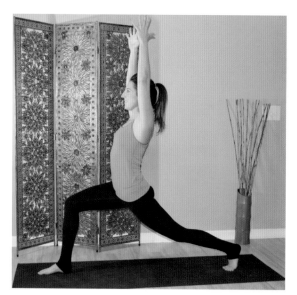

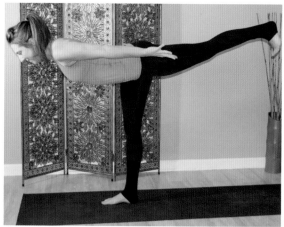

Eagle with Forward Fold

Bring your hands together at your heart. Bend your knees and hinge at your hips. Slowly lift your right leg up and over your left, crossing at the thighs and below the knees. Reach your arms forward and wrap your right arm under the left at your elbows. Cross again to bring your hands to touch. Hold for three breaths and release to a forward fold. Hold for five breaths and repeat on the opposite side.

Boat Series

Boat Pose
Table Top
Boat

From your forward fold, walk your feet out to the edges of your mat. Turn your toes out to the side slightly. Squat down and bring your hands together at your heart. Lift your chest as you sink your hips down toward

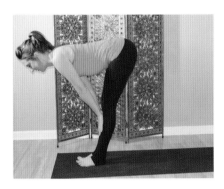

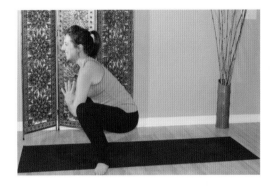

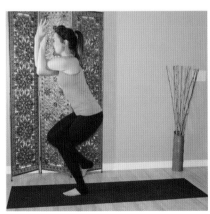

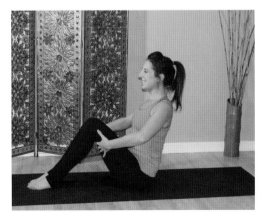

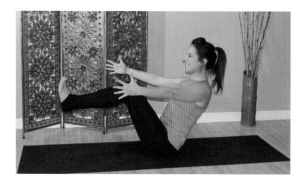

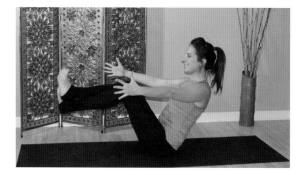

lengthened and your core engaged. Hold for 3 breaths. Cross your right ankle over your left and draw your heel in toward you. Rock forward and plant your hands on the mat. Step your feet back to downward dog.

Downward Facing Dog to Pigeon
Reach your right leg behind you as high as you can. Slowly bring it forward, placing your right knee outside of your right wrist and your shin across, at an angle, to the left side of your mat. Lengthen your left leg down the mat behind you and drop your pelvis as close to the ground as possible, without leaning to the right or left. Stay centered over your pelvis as your lengthen your spine and then fold forward over your right leg. Hold for ten breaths.

the ground. Place your elbows on the insides of your knees to press the groin open. Hold for three breaths. Reach your hands behind you and gently sit down onto your mat. Bring the soles of your feet to the ground and hold on to the back of your thighs. Lift your chest and engage your belly button into your spine. Slowly lift your heels. Hold for one breath. Flex your feet to lift your toes and balance. Slowly reach your heels forward and up until your shins are parallel to the mat. Reach our arms out to the sides for boat pose. Keep your spine

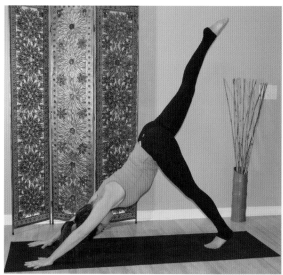

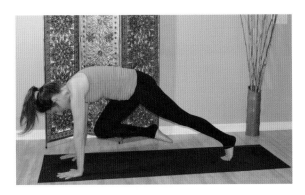

Half Fold to Twist

Walk your hands back to lift your torso. Shift to your right hip and sweep your left leg around to the front. Cross it over your right leg into a twist. Reach your left hand behind you to lengthen your spine and wrap your right arm around your left knee to twist deeper. Hold for three breaths.

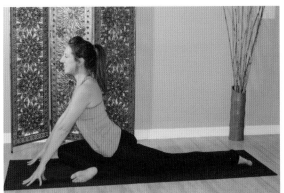

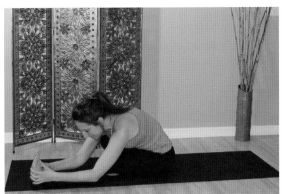

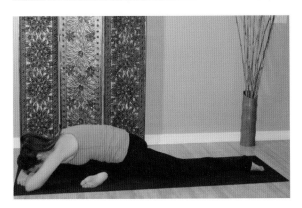

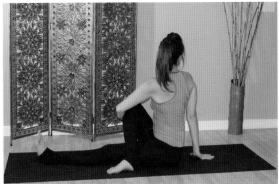

Double Pigeon, Table Top, and Boat Pose
Slowly unwind to the center. Bring your shins parallel, stacking the left leg on top of the right. Your knees and ankles will stack here to keep your shins parallel like firelogs. Lift your heart and slowly fold forward, keeping your spine lengthened. Hold for five breaths. After five breaths, release your legs, bringing the soles of your feet to the mat, hips distance apart. Slide your hands behind you with your fingertips pointing toward you. Push into your hands and feet to press your hips up into a reverse table top position. Hold for two breaths and release. Take boat pose and repeat the entire sequence on the opposite side, ending again in boat pose.

Seated Series

Seated Fold to Roll Down
Stretch your legs out in front of you. Squeeze them together and sit with a tall spine. Place your hands next to your hips to help lengthen. Slowly lean forward, hinging from your hips, into seated forward fold. Flex your feet and reach toward your shins or toes. Hold for five breaths. Slowly point your toes, draw your belly button into your spine and roll down onto the mat, letting each part of your back touch down as you roll down.

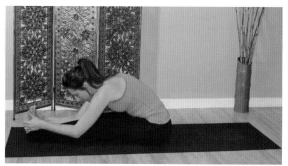

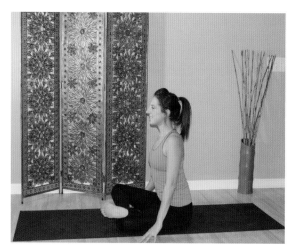

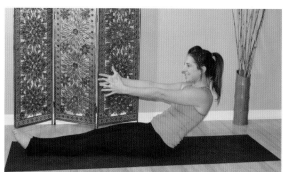

Shoulderstand to Plow Pose

Bring your knees into your chest and slowly reach your toes behind your head. Place your hands on your lower back with your elbows close together. Lift your legs toward the ceiling and slide your arms farther down your back. Hold for five breaths. Slowly release your toes down to the ground behind your head into plow pose. If they touch down, release your hands. If they hover above the ground, keep your hands on your back. Hold for three breaths.

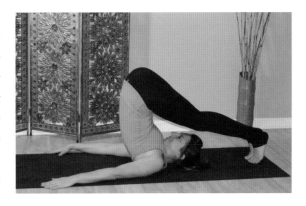

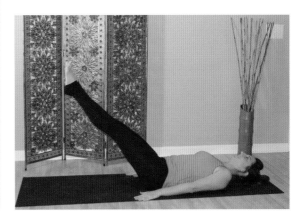

Fish Pose to Reclined Twist

Roll down your spine, using your hands and core as brakes, and lengthen your legs all the way onto your mat. Slide your hands under your thighs, push onto your elbows, and lift your chest, head, and upper arms off the mat. Arch your chest and touch the crown of your head down to the ground for fish pose. Hold for three breaths and release by tucking your chin and lowering down. Hug your knees into your chest. Reach your arms out to a "T" and drop your knees over to the right side. Turn your head and gaze to the left. Hold for five breaths. Repeat on the opposite side.

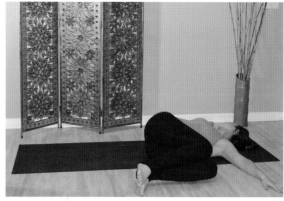

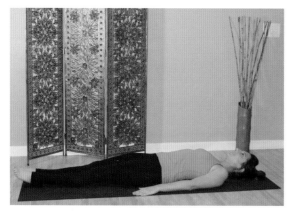

Happy Baby Pose

Hug your knees back into your chest. Reach through your knees and grab your big toes. Open the toes and knees wide as your draw your knees toward your shoulders in happy baby. Hold for three breaths. Release your knees back into your chest. Slowly lower all the way down to lie flat on your mat.

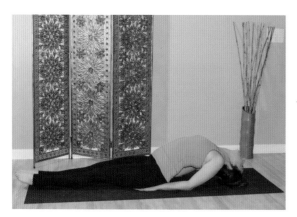

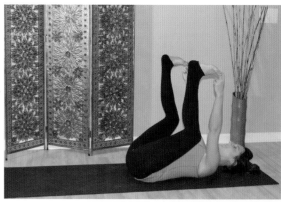

Savasana

Let your feet stretch out to the corners of your mat. Bring your hands down by your sides, slightly away from your body with your palms facing up. Slightly tuck your chin to release the back of your neck. Close your eyes. Take a deep breath in and hold it. Open your mouth and exhale to release. Hold here for at least five minutes. Stay still with your body. Let your breath fall in and out naturally. And let any thought simply come in and drift away. After at least five minutes, start to wiggle your fingers and toes. Roll your wrists and ankles. Reach your arms up over head and stretch from fingertips to toes. Roll onto your right side, bending you knees and making a pillow with your arms. Slowly roll up to a cross-legged position. Place your hands together at your heart and keep your eyes closed. Hold for five breaths, soaking in the balance and space after your practice. Namaste.

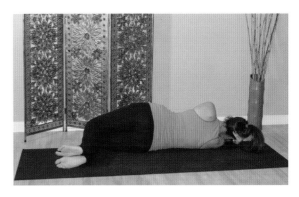

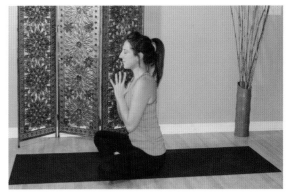

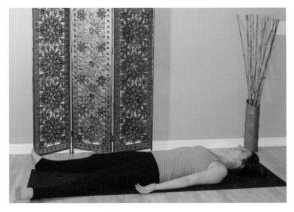

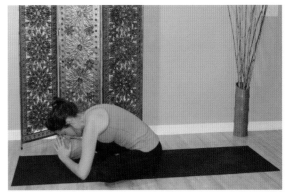

STRETCHY YOGA

Hold each stretch for two minutes unless otherwise specified.

Child's Pose

Sit on your heels with your knees wide and your big toes together. Lower your chest down to the ground and stretch your arms forward. Try to keep your hips on your heels.

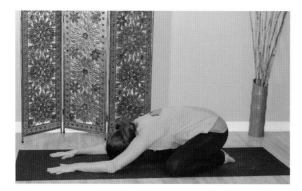

Downward-Facing Dog *(hold for five breaths)*

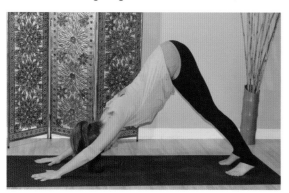

Tuck your toes and straighten your legs as you lift your hips up to downward-facing dog. Spread your fingers wide and press your heels down to the ground. Squeeze your thighs to help lengthen your legs.

Rag Doll *(hold for five breaths)*

From downward dog, walk your feet forward to the top of the mat. Separate your feet to the edges of the mat and hang down, letting your head and neck release. Grab opposite elbows and sway from side to side to help release tension in your back.

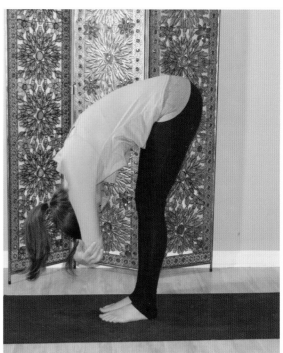

Mountain Pose (*hold for five breaths*)
Slowly roll up your spine to standing. Roll your shoulders up, back, and down to open your chest. Bring your hands to your heart and close your eyes.

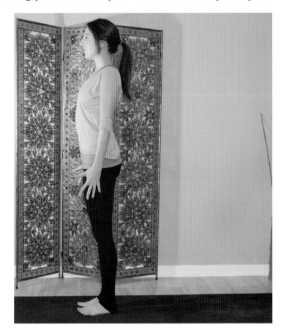

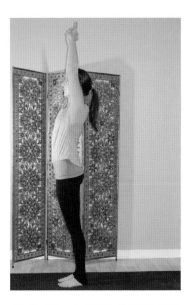

Extended Reach and Half Moon (*hold for five breaths on each side*)
Reach your arms up overhead and clasp your hands. Bring your palms together as you extend your index fingers. Keep your shoulder blades sliding down your back as you extend your elbows and lean to the right. Roll your chest up and open to the left slightly. Inhale to come back up and repeat on the opposite side.

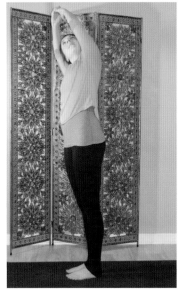

Wide-Footed Forward Fold (*hold for five breaths*)
Bring your feet to the edges of the mat. Release your hands and reach them out to the sides as you fold forward. Wrap your hands behind you knees and hold on to opposite elbows or forearms.

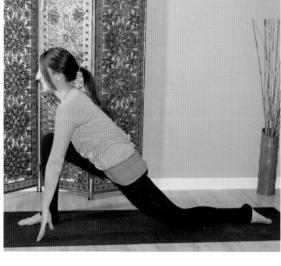

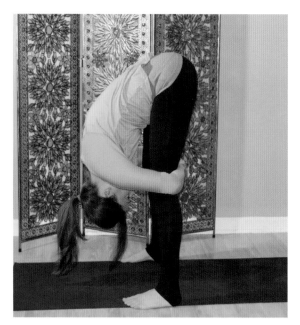

Low Lunge
Step your left leg back down the mat as far as you can. Bend your right knee over your ankle and lower your left knee to the mat, untucking your toes. Press your hips forward toward your right heel and reach your arms up toward the ceiling.

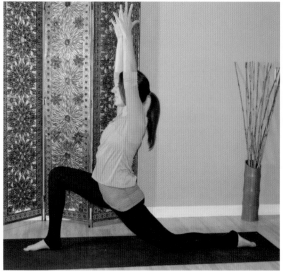

Half Hanumanasana

Bring your hands down on either side of your foot. Straighten your front leg and send your hips back, sitting your right hip above your right heel. Flex your right foot and fold over your right leg.

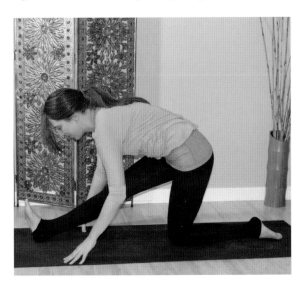

Pigeon Pose

Move back to your low lunge. Wiggle your right leg across your mat until your shin is almost parallel to the front of the mat. Lower your pelvis down toward the mat and fold over your shin. Step back to downward dog. Walk your hands back and lift your torso. Tuck your back toes under and lift your knee. Step back to downward dog. Press both heels toward the ground and then walk your feet to your hands.

From downward dog, lower your knees to child's pose. See above to repeat sequence on the opposite side.

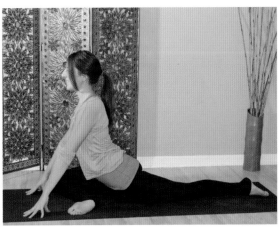

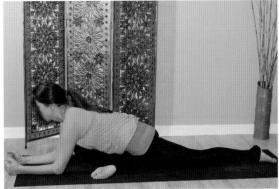

Camel Pose (*hold for five breaths*)

Come to stand on your knees and tuck your toes under. You can roll up the mat or place a blanket under your knees if the ground is too hard. Bring your hands to your lower back with your fingertips reaching up. Draw your elbows in to engage the sides of the body and open your heart. Press your hips forward and draw your navel in toward your spine. Lift your rib cage off your waist and reach your heart up toward the ceiling. If you are comfortable here, reach for your heels and lift even higher. To come out of the pose, bring your hands back to your lower back and engage your core as you slowly rise back up.

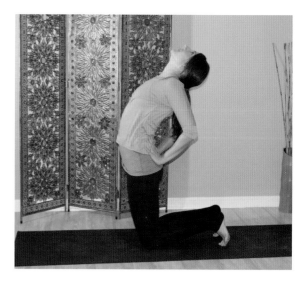

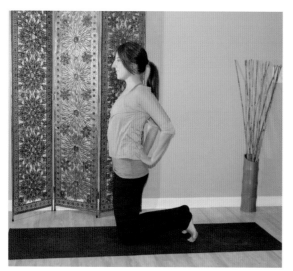

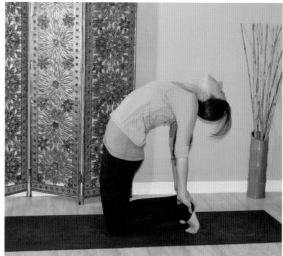

Hero's Pose with Alternate Nostril Breathing (*hold for ten breaths*)

Sit on your heels with the toes released. Bring your palms onto your thighs and lengthen your spine. Bring your right hand to your nose. Inhale and place your thumb over your right nostril. Exhale and inhale through your left side. Place your ring finger over your left nostril, release the thumb, and exhale/inhale out the right. Repeat this breath for five rounds (ten breaths total).

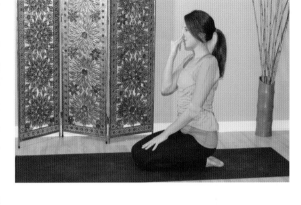

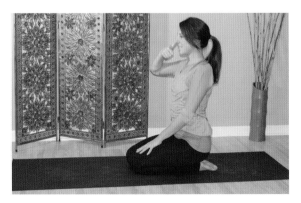

Seated Forward Fold

Bring your legs out in front of you. Flex your feet and sit as tall as you can. If you feel rounded through your spine or your tailbone feels tucked, sit on a blanket or pillow. Lengthen your spine and slowly fold over your legs, bringing your chest toward your shins and your gaze at your ankles. If your arms are near your toes, you can hold on to the feet.

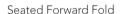

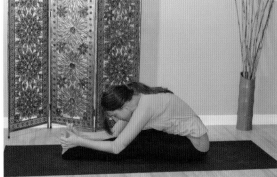

Wide-Legged Fold

Lift back up and open the legs as wide as you can. Keep your feet flexed. Lengthen your spine and fold forward. Your hands can reach forward or toward your toes. If you feel stuck or are unable to fold, bring your hands behind you and press into your fingertips to help lengthen the spine and create space.

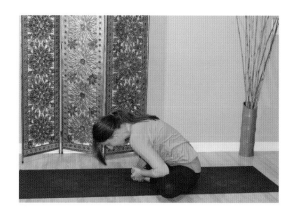

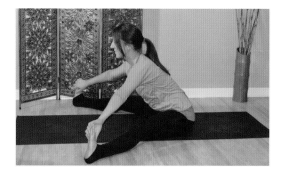

Cobblers Pose

Bring the soles of your feet together and clasp your hands around your feet. Use this grip to lengthen your spine and fold forward, leading with your chest.

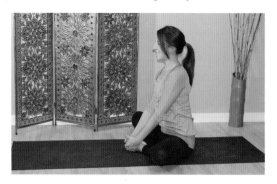

Knees to Chest

Lift back up to a seated position and draw your knees together. Slowly roll down onto your back. Hug your knees into your chest and make tiny circles to each side to release your spine.

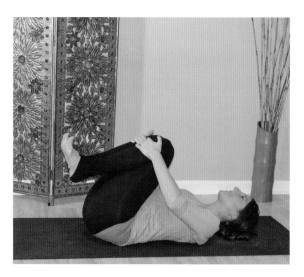

Legs Up the Wall

Bring your feet down to the ground. Lift your hips slightly and slide a pillow, folded blanket, or yoga block under your sacrum. Lift your legs up to the ceiling. Your arms can rest out to the sides or on your belly.

the mat and flex your foot. Twist your right knee across your body to the left. Reach your right arm out to the right side. Repeat on the opposite side.

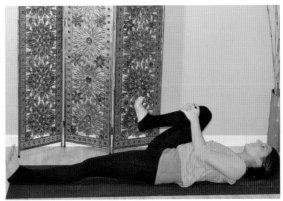

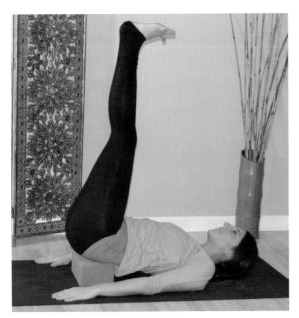

Single Leg Twist (*hold for ten breaths*)

Lower your legs to remove your prop and hug your knees into your chest. Release your left leg down to

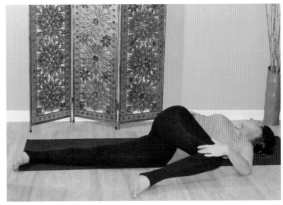

Happy Baby

Hug your knees into your chest. Reach through your knees and grab onto your big toes. Open your feet and knees wide as you draw your knees toward your shoulders. You can rock slightly side to side here to release the lower back.

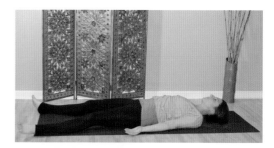

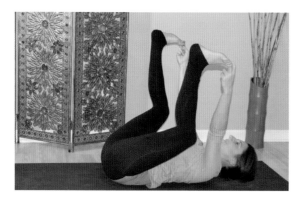

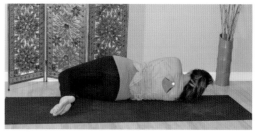

Savasana *(hold for five minutes)*

Hug your knees back into your chest. Lower all the way down to the ground. Separate your feet out to the corners of your mat and let the feet fall open. Bring your hands down by your sides away from the body with your palms facing up. Slightly tuck your chin and close your eyes. Try to let any tension in the body or thoughts in the mind pass by. Stay here for at least five minutes. After five minutes, reach your arms up over head. Roll onto your right side, bending your knees and making a pillow with your arms. Slowly roll up to a comfortable seated position with your eyes closed. Bring your hands together at your heart. Namaste.

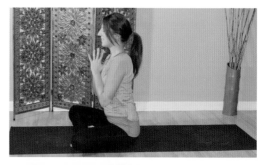

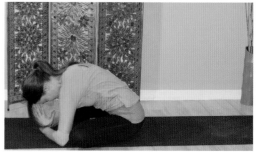

Chapter Five: Weekly Meal Plans

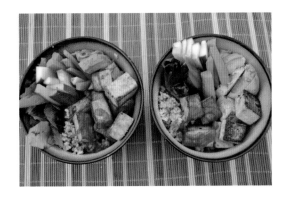

Throughout the next three weeks, you'll be changing the way you eat to clean up your system, restore your digestion, and improve your energy. You'll start with the one-day juice cleanse, slowly move into eating raw foods, and by the end of the week incorporate low-acidic, whole, unprocessed foods. You'll feel full, satisfied, and energized without feeling deprived.

Below is a suggested meal plan for the next twenty-one days, which includes three meals and three snacks a day. You may not need to eat all of these snacks, or you may feel that some days you need a little more. This is OK, just stick to the "Do's and Don'ts" guideline outlined for you earlier in the book. Try to stick with mostly raw snacks and remember you can drink all the juice you would like.

Each day, with each meal, drink at least one glass of water. Continue drinking water and/or herbal tea, such as the detox tea or hot lemon water, throughout the day to help flush toxins out of your system and keep you hydrated as you exercise.

You'll also start each day with Hot Lemon Water as outlined in your daily routine.

	Monday	Tuesday	Wednesday	Thursday	Friday	Saturday	Sunday
Week 1	Basic Green Juice	Detox Beet Juice	Go Green Juice	Root Veg Juice	Green Zinger	Green and Clean Smoothie	Go Green Juice
	Strawberry Fields Juice	*Avocado*	*Apple or other Fruit*	*Carrot and Date Bowl (NO nuts!)*	*Carrot and Date Bowl w/Nuts*	*Avocado*	*Vegan Overnight Oats*
	Detox Beet Juice	Green Smoothie	Handful Mixed Greens, Carrot Ginger Soup	Sweet Potato Fries and Mixed Greens	Red, White, and Blue Salad	Mango Salad	Black Bean Bowl
	Cool Down Juice	*3–5 Dates*	*Green Zinger*	*Cucumber slices or other vegetables*	*Green Lemonade Juice*	*Apple Slices and Raw Almond Butter*	*Strawberry Fields Juice*
	Green and Clean Juice	Carrot and Ginger Soup, Handful of Spring Mix	Simple greens and mixed greens	Sauteed Kale and brown rice with mixed greens	Mango Buddha Bowl	Brussels Sprouts and Tofu Bowl	Sweet Potato Fries, Sauteed Kale, Green Juice
	Green Lemonade Juice	*Banana Soft Serve*	*Avocado*	*Strawberry Fields Juice*	*Banana Soft Serve*	*Basic Green Juice*	*2 Energy Balls*

	Monday	Tuesday	Wednesday	Thursday	Friday	Saturday	Sunday
Week 2	Basic Green Juice	Green Detox Smoothie	Green and Clean Juice	Root Veg Juice	Green Detox Smoothie	Basic Green Juice	Red Raspberry Smoothie
	Superfood Chocolate Bar	*Apple Cinnamon Bars*	*Apples and Almond Butter*	*Carrot and Date Bowl*	*Detox Beet Juice*	*Vegan Overnight Oats*	*Almond Butter Dates*
	Taste the Rainbow Salad	Detox Kale Salad	Black Bean Stuffed Avocado	Taste the Rainbow Salad	Chickpea and Cucumber Bowl	Butternut Squash Soup	Detox Kale Salad
	Strawberry Fields Juice	*Raw Veggies and Nuts*	*2 Energy Balls*	*Green Zinger*	*Almond Butter Date Bites*	*Green Lemonade*	*Avocado*
	Chickpea Taco Bowl	Sautéed Brussels and Grains	Chickpea and Beet Bowl	Kale and Tomatoes with Brown Rice	Butternut Squash Soup and Mixed Greens	Spicy Tofu Bowl for Two	Tempeh Scramble
	Almond Butter Dates	*Popcorn*	*Berry Ice Cream*	*Superfood Chocolate Bar*	*Popcorn*	*Berry Ice Cream*	*Superfood Chocolate Bar*

	Monday	Tuesday	Wednesday	Thursday	Friday	Saturday	Sunday
Week 3	Gorgeously Green Smoothie *2 Energy Balls* Carrot Ginger Soup and ½ avocado *Cool Down Juice* Spicy Tofu Bowl for Two *Apple Slices and Almond Butter*	Green and Clean Juice *Apple Cinnamon Bars* Black Bean Stuffed Avocados *Veggies and Nuts* Kale and Tomatoes with brown rice or grains *Berry Ice Cream*	Blueberry Magic Smoothie *2 Energy Balls* Carrot Ginger Soup w/Avocado *Green Zinger Juice* Chickpea Taco Bowl *Banana Soft Serve*	Go Green Juice *Almond Butter Date Bites* Chickpea and Cucumber Salad *Veggies and Nuts* Sauteed Brussels Sprouts, Quinoa, Mixed Greens *Superfood Chocolate Bar*	Detox Beet Juice *Vegan Overnight Oats* Detox Kale Salad *Red Raspberry Smoothie* Black Bean Bowl *2 Energy Balls*	Go Green Juice *Apple Slices and Almond Butter* Mango Buddha Bowl *Dates* Butternut Squash Soup *Superfood Chocolate Bar*	Basic Green Juice *Avocado* Red and Blue Salad *Apple Slices and Almond Butter* Tempeh Scramble *Berry Ice Cream*

Chapter Six: Week One: Intense Clean-Up and Rest

This first week is all about unplugging a bit to recharge. You'll start off with a one-day juice/smoothie/soup (pureed or broth) cleanse to give your digestive system a break, release toxins, and flush them out of your system. Then throughout the week, you'll slowly add foods back in. Start by adding in raw foods as snacks. Maybe a few cucumber or carrot sticks, a sliced apple, or a smoothie. Then you'll start cooking your veggies but remain grain-free for another day. After that, you can experiment with wheat- and gluten-free grains, such as quinoa, millet, amaranth, and rice. After that, you can start adding in beans, nuts, and legumes.

Each day will start with a fresh green juice or smoothie and will contain unprocessed, minimally packaged foods. Think lots of fresh produce, whole grains, and raw nuts. You will be eating cooked veggies and grains, but shoot for a fresh juice or salad with each meal if the meal itself is not raw.

When you eat a highly nutritious diet, with lots of nutrients per bite, there is no need to count calories, carbs, or protein. Your body will be getting plenty of all of these. And if you feel hungry, snack on more veggies! So really, don't worry about protein in this first week. You'll be eating mostly green, leafy veggies, which are actually high in protein. And most of these wheat-free grains are also high in protein. In fact, quinoa is one of the only plant-based complete proteins.

Also, you might be cutting way back on exercise this week. If you are a gym-rat or marathoner of any kind, you may feel a little uneasy to know that in this first week, exercise is a minimum. But no worries, there is a good reason for it. As mentioned before, too much exercise can cause an acidic, inflammatory reaction in the body, which is the exact opposite of what we want to create when cleansing. We are also highly changing the diet, and it can be exhausting for the body to get used to in the first few days. By taking exercise slowly and gently, you can support your cleanse without depleting your energy.

In this first week, you'll try a few simple yoga poses and routines. You'll start with a few sun-salutations, a few gentle twists, and deep folds to hold for a few minutes each. Next week you'll add a few light—three pounds or less—weights. You want to make sure that you keep your body moving, but in a soothing, gentle way. The aim here is not to burn calories but to help flush out toxins and keep your digestive system moving.

EXERCISE

Slow it down is your motto this week. It might seem counterproductive to exercise less on a cleanse, but your body will need rest, especially in the beginning. Now this doesn't mean you'll be sedentary. You'll just be moving in ways that really benefit the detoxification process and support you mentally.

FOOD

There are no specific food guidelines that you have to go by every day, but there is a suggested meal plan for you to follow to help reduce the stress of planning. This plan features many of the recipes also featured later in the book. You can use these each day for the optimal detox, but if you aren't able to get some of these foods or feel like trying your own recipe, go for it! Just stick to the foods on your do's and don'ts list and get creative!

DAY ONE: LIQUID CLEANSE

MOTTO OF THE DAY

"Every journey begins with a single step."

Day one starts off the deep cleansing portion of your three weeks. In this first day, you'll stick to a liquid and/or pureed diet. This way, the food has already been broken down a bit through juicing or blending, and it is easier for the nutrients to be absorbed into your system. It also gives the digestive system a little break, because some of the work is already done to release digestive enzymes and process your food.

If you stick to liquid juices, rather than smoothies or pureed soups, you'll get these benefits even more. When you juice, the fiber—which is the harder, slower part to digest—is removed, so you are able to absorb the nutrients almost immediately into your bloodstream and organs. If you have smoothies or soups, it just takes a little longer, but not as long as it would with solid food.

There are three levels to this day. You can juice fast, juice and smoothie fast, or have juices/smoothies/pureed soups. Decide which level you need to be at and consider this the first "exercise" in tuning in to what your body needs.

The juicing is the most restrictive of the three diets, but again, it gives your system the biggest break and the most immediate nutrients. If you have a juicer available, I highly recommend this one. Shoot for three large (pint size) juices and three smaller (half pint) juices today. If you need more, go ahead and have a few more.

If you are unable to juice or purchase fresh juices (not the stuff on the supermarket shelves), and only have access to a blender, smoothies and soups are perfectly fine. Just add your ingredients in and blend away. Stick to veggies, some fruits, and unsweetened non-dairy milk for these smoothies.

For your soups, steam your vegetables, as this allows for the least amount of enzymes to be killed off in the cooking process. Then add it to the blender with a little water and blend until smooth.

Remember that all of these should be made fresh. No store bought juices, smoothies, or soups unless you know they are freshly made and unpasteurized. We want them to be minimally cooked with the most nutrition available.

You may notice today some frustration as you get hungry. You may also start to have some detox symptoms such as a headache, indigestion, or upset stomach. All of these are perfectly normal and part of the cleanse. They will slowly get better after a day or two.

As far as digestion goes, you may be heading to the restroom a bit more today to "flush" out your toxins, or you may feel a bit sluggish. Again, both are normal, it just depends on how your body reacts to the cleanse. Either way, make sure you drink plenty of water to help aide in the flushing out of toxins.

DAILY FOCUS

"I already have everything I need within me."

It is very easy for us to get caught up in wanting results instantaneously. The truth is, though, that lasting change takes hard work and time. As you begin your journey back to health and happiness today, remember that it takes one step at a time to get down your path, and you already have all the tools you need to make it through these next few weeks. Allow this thought to be your guide throughout the day. When you get stressed, when you get hungry, when you feel healthy, and when you feel like you want to give up—this is your reminder to keep you motivated. You don't have to be perfect today or ever. It's all part of the journey that starts today and you have everything you need within you.

Take a few moments (about five minutes) in the morning and evening and sit quietly with your intention. Start by closing your eyes and breathing in and out for five counts each. Repeat this for ten rounds, until the breath flows in and out with ease. If sitting with your eyes closed is too much, you can always sit and focus on one particular object.

Keep your gaze focused, eyes opened or closed, and simply repeat your mantra for the five minutes. Afterward, jot down any feelings, thoughts, or goals that have come up for you with your mantra today.

POSE OF THE DAY

Today your pose will focus on helping you coax along your detox with a forward fold. Forward folds will help support your system in three ways. Physically, the folding motion compresses digestive organs, so they are squeezed and "wrung out." This helps to push any released toxins through your system. Forward folds are also very calming for the body. This calming sensation can help to decrease any stress you may be feeling. These folds will also help you to cool down your body and mind, helping decrease inflammation. Sit with your legs stretched out and your feet flexed. Lengthen your spine by sitting tall. Hinge from your hips and drape over your legs. Try to aim the chest toward your shins. If needed, place a pillow or bolster on your legs to drape onto. Hold this pose for 3 to 5 minutes.

*Tip: When you hold your pose, try not to hold your breath. This is a great time to practice breathing in and out for five counts.

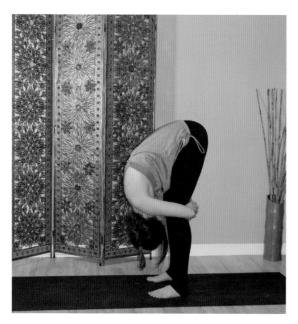

Sitting/Standing Forward Fold

SELF-CARE TIP OF THE DAY

Hot Water with Lemon

Before you eat or drink anything today, even a glass of cool water, drink a mug of hot water with lemon. The enzymes in the lemon help to kick-start your digestion for the day, and the water helps to rehydrate you, flush toxins from your system, and keep your digestive system moving along. You'll do this today, and continue it each day during the cleanse. Warm a mug of water until almost boiling. Squeeze the juice of one small lemon (or half a large lemon) into your mug. Mix together and drink.

DAILY ROUTINE

Today you begin the journey to regain your health and happiness.

- On your first day, start by taking a deep breath. You have everything within you to make it through the next few weeks. It's not about perfection. It's about taking time to tune in to you and make a commitment to finding happiness through better health.
- Head to the kitchen and make some warm water with lemon juice. Drink this first to get your digestion going to wake up your digestion and your system as you start the day.
- Next head to your meditation station.
- After meditation, if there is time, try out pose of the day, self-care tip, and your daily exercise practice.
- Go ahead and start your daily routine. Make some juice for your first meal, juice for your morning snack, and more juice throughout the day. Drink plenty of water, herbal tea, and hot lemon water throughout the day.
- At the end of your day, meditate again and see how the mantra might sit differently with you now. Practice your self-care tip and pose, and exercise if you haven't already.
- At the end of the night, head to bed and settle in for seven to nine hours of sleep. Before drifting off, give yourself a high five or a bear hug for making it through the first day safe and sound.

DAY TWO: ADD IN RAW FOODS

MOTTO OF THE DAY

"The only thing that stands between you and your dream is the will to try and the belief that it is actually possible." —Joel Brown

You've made it through your first Congratulations!

On the second day, you have already released many toxins into your system, and right now they are trying to figure out how to get out of your body. This is a very good thing, but it doesn't always feel so good. Today, or maybe even tomorrow, you might start to feel a little, well, yucky. You might have a headache, an upset stomach, feel sluggish or tired, or maybe even feel like you have the flu. This is normal, and it will pass. Rest and drink water, or maybe try some hot water with a squeeze of lemon. Sit down and meditate. Move your body and breathe deeply.

Keep going and know that a little hard work and a little sacrifice can take you leaps and bounds toward your health and happiness goals. Stay strong. You've got this!

Today you'll slowly add in raw, whole foods to your diet. These foods will be simple, fresh, and highly nutritious. These will be the easiest for your body to digest after a liquid feast, and they are full of digestive enzymes and nutrients to continue flushing out your system. Keep drinking juice with your raw meals or as a snack in between. Start small though. If you rush into eating a large portion of food after a liquid break, you may notice a lot of digestive discomfort, heaviness, and bloating. Stick to eating a few pieces of fruits and veggies as snacks.

You'll start off again with a fresh juice or smoothie. If you feel hungry for a snack, try a piece of fresh fruit or a vegetable. A half of an avocado makes a nice, creamy snack mid-morning. For lunch, try a pureed soup or another smoothie. Again, you can snack on fresh fruits or veggies as needed. For dinner, a soup or smoothie is fine, but pair it with a light salad, full of raw vegetables or fruit. For your dressing, try a drizzle of olive oil and half a squeezed lemon.

You can have an additional raw snack after your dinner.

DAILY FOCUS

"I have it within me right now to get me where I want to be later."

Today, you may notice your will wavering a bit. The excitement might be wearing off, or perhaps you aren't feeling so great. But keep your focus into the future a bit. This moment will pass and you will feel better soon. A detox doesn't last forever, but the tools you learn along the way do.

Take five minutes in the morning and evening to sit with your mantra. Recite it, ponder it, and let it flow through you as your motivation for the day.

POSE OF THE DAY

Today your pose will focus on helping you coax along your detox with twists. Twists also help move toxins through the body by wringing out your organs and pushing toxins through your system. Today, we'll also add a bit of breath work in with your pose to give you the added benefits of deep, powerful, calming breath with a twisting detox.

Sit in a cross-legged position. Inhale and reach your arms overhead. Exhale as you twist to your right,

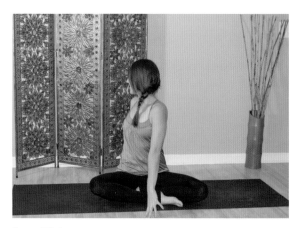

Seated Twist

bringing your right hand behind you and your left hand across your right thigh. Inhale and reach your arms up as you turn back to the center. Exhale to twist to the left. Repeat this ten times on each side. After you finish, sit still and close your eyes. Just take a moment to notice your breath moving in and out, strong and steady.

SELF-CARE TIP OF THE DAY

Tongue Scraping

*You'll need a metal (or plastic if that is all you can find) tongue scraper, which can be purchased at a local pharmacy or health food store. They are fairly inexpensive. This will be a worthwhile investment for your health and you'll use it each morning (and night) of your detox.

Before brushing your teeth, use your tongue scraper to remove unhealthy bacteria and residue from your tongue. This will help stimulate digestion, which begins in your mouth. Your saliva and good bacteria work to break down your food, making the digestive enzymes more readily available. When you scrape your tongue, you clear away the bad bacteria and residue that build up while you sleep and make room for the good bacteria and saliva to start working.

Simply reach the scraper straight back on your tongue and pull it forward to scrape. Release and repeat along the left and right sides of the roof of your tongue.

DAILY ROUTINE

Today you practice tapping into your willpower at your center.

- On your second day start by taking a deep breath into the belly. Exhale and open your mouth to release any tension, negativity, or funk that might have built up overnight. Remember, today might be tough, but you have the willpower within you to stick to it.

- Get up and get going. Brush your teeth and scrape your tongue using a metal tongue scraper. This will help you remove unwanted bacteria from your tongue, leave your breath a little fresher, and start to stimulate digestion. All of which will help you feel more bright and shiny today, instead of feeling funky and cranky.

- Head to the kitchen and make some warm water with lemon juice. Drink this first to wake up your digestive system and energize you as you start the day.

- Next head to your meditation station. Set a timer for five minutes. In your meditation, sit and silently repeat your daily motto. At the end of the five minutes, try your breath and pose of the day. If there is time, practice your exercise of the day.

- Go ahead and start your daily routine. Make some juice for your first meal. If you are feeling extra famished, light-headed, or even a bit weak, make a smoothie instead or pair your juice with an avocado half or pureed carrots and dates.

- For a mid-morning snack, have a piece of raw fruit or vegetable. The other avocado half also works well in the morning.
- Have lunch around 12 p.m.
- For a mid-afternoon snack, keep it raw or pureed again. Smoothies, fruits, and vegetables all work great for a mid-afternoon boost.
- *Optional time to exercise if not done in the morning.
- For dinner, incorporate more solid food, such as a raw salad with soup. Try to have dinner between 6 and 7 p.m.
- You can have another raw snack after dinner.
- Drink plenty of water, herbal tea, and hot lemon water throughout the day. This will help to keep your digestive system flowing and your skin glowing.
- Before bed, meditate again and see how the mantra might sit differently with you now. Practice your self-care tip and pose if you haven't already.
- At the end of the night, head to bed and settle in for seven to nine hours of sleep. Before drifting off, tell yourself one thing you are proud of accomplishing on your second day.

DAY THREE: ADD IN COOKED VEGGIES

MOTTO OF THE DAY

"Belief overflows to behavior. First we need to change what we believe. When we truly change what we believe, we'll gladly change how we behave." —Craig Groeschel, *Soul Detox*

On day three, let the cooking begin! You've given your body some time to recuperate from the first-day cleanse, so now it's time to add in some cooked vegetables. To keep it simple, you'll stick to cooking, and mostly steaming, vegetables today in addition to your raw produce, juices, and smoothies. Steaming allows you to cook your vegetables without boiling out the nutrients. Plus, steaming your veggies is a huge timesaver. You can have them steaming in a pot while you read a book, finish some chores, or practice your pose of the day. And since it keeps a good deal of the nutrients intact, you'll know you are absorbing more health with each bite. Sautéing is also good for today and is a timesaver, because most veggies require little time to sauté and are even quite tasty when they are still a bit crisp or, in fancy terms, al dente.

Remember to add in raw juices or salads with your cooked meal to help increase the digestive enzymes and fresh nutrients you are receiving.

Experiment with all kinds of vegetables, but focus largely on leafy greens, including lettuces, kale, broccoli, and spinach. These have the most nutrients per bite.

Try steaming some broccoli and topping it with nutritional yeast, or sauté some kale with onions and garlic. And with each meal, add a little green juice and raw salad on the side for added enzymes. Even a handful of mixed greens will do the trick.

DAILY FOCUS

"I believe in my power to make the change."

There are times when we can become our own worst enemy. When we are hot and agitated or working through a stressful time, the negativity in our own mind starts to grow louder. As you move through your detox, there may be moments, especially in the beginning, where this voice is raging, yelling at you each and every moment. But if you take it back to the positive, you can clear this voice away.

In your meditation, and throughout the day today, come back to your belief in yourself, even if it is unsteady. Convince yourself by repeating to yourself, "I believe in my power to make the change." You'll find that the more you say it, the more you truly believe it.

And as you start to believe it, it opens the gates for calm and peaceful space within your body and mind.

Take five minutes in the morning and evening to sit with your mantra. Recite it, ponder it, and let it flow through you as your motivation for the day.

POSE OF THE DAY

Stand with your feet together and your hands on your hips. Step your left foot back about three feet and turn

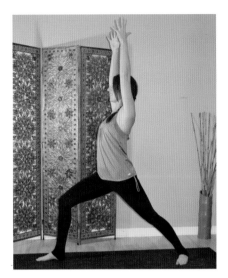

Warrior I

your toes out slightly. Press your left foot into the mat by squeezing your thigh and pressing into your heel. Bend your right knee over your ankle and engage your inner thighs to keep your hip facing forward as much as possible. Stretch your arms up by your ears and reach for the ceiling. Draw your shoulder-blades down your back and turn your palms to face in toward each other. Hold for five breaths and then switch sides.

SELF-CARE TIP OF THE DAY

Alternate Nostril Breathing

This helps to balance the right and left sides of the body, calm your nervous system, and clear out any fogginess in your mind.

Sit with your legs crossed. Bring your right hand to your nose. You'll use your thumb and ring finger for this exercise. Let your first two fingers rest on between your eyebrows on your "third eye." Inhale through both nostrils. Plug your right nostril with your thumb and exhale/inhale through the left. Release your thumb and plug the left nostril with your ring finger. Exhale/inhale through your right. Repeat this ten times. After the tenth time, release and exhale through both nostrils.

DAILY ROUTINE

- On your third day start by taking a deep breath into the belly and stretching from your fingers to toes to wake your body. Exhale and open your mouth to release any tension, negativity, or funk that might have built up overnight.
- Get up and get going. Brush your teeth and scrape your tongue using a metal tongue scraper. This will help you remove unwanted bacteria from your tongue, leave your breath a little fresher, and start to stimulate digestion. All of which will help you feel more bright and shiny today, instead of feeling funky and cranky.
- Head to the kitchen and make some warm water with lemon juice. Drink this first to wake up your digestive system and energize you as you start the day.
- Next head to your meditation station. Set a timer for five minutes. In your meditation, sit and silently repeat your daily motto. At the end of the five minutes, try your breath and pose of the day. If there is time, give your self-care tip a try and practice your exercise of the day.
- Go ahead and start your daily routine. Make some juice for your first meal. If you are feeling extra famished, light-headed, or even a bit weak, make a smoothie instead or pair your juice with an avocado half or pureed carrots and dates. You might even want to try some steamed or sautéed veggies as part of your breakfast or morning snack today. Asparagus, kale, and spinach all make delicious, flavorful, and detoxifying green morning additions.
- For a mid-morning snack, have a piece of raw fruit or vegetable. The other avocado half also works well in the morning.
- Have lunch around 12 p.m. If you have cooked vegetables, add in a small raw greens salad. These enzymes will help you digest and keep releasing toxins.
- For a mid-afternoon snack, smoothies, juices, fruits, and vegetables all work great for an energy boost.
- *Optional time to exercise if not done in morning.
- For dinner, incorporate more steamed and raw foods, such as a raw salad with soup or steamed vegetables. Try to have dinner between 6 and 7 p.m.
- You can have another raw snack after dinner.

- Drink plenty of water, herbal tea, and hot lemon water throughout the day. This will help to keep your digestive system flowing and your skin glowing.
- Before bed, meditate again and see how the mantra might sit differently with you now. Practice your self-care tip and pose if you haven't already. At the end of the night, head to bed and settle in for seven to nine hours of sleep. Before drifting off, tell yourself one thing you are proud of accomplishing on your third day.

DAY FOUR: ADD IN GRAINS

MOTTO OF THE DAY

"Don't judge each day by the harvest you reap but by the seeds that you plant." —Robert Louis Stevenson

On the fourth day, you can begin eating grains again. After eating just fruits, vegetables, and juices for a few days, you may feel in need of some variety and something more substantial. Today we start to add in healthy, whole grains to your diet. For these grains, you'll want to keep them wheat- and gluten-free. Gluten and wheat are often culprits of stomach issues and inflammation. Even if you are not allergic, you might still have trouble digesting them. Look for gluten in breads, pastas, and also in seitan, a wheat meat alternative.

Quinoa, amaranth, millet, oatmeal, and rice are all acceptable to eat during the cleanse, starting on day four. These whole grains are high in fiber and protein and contain many nutrients. They keep you feeling full, give you energy, and support your system during your cleanse. Try cooking them the same way you would cook regular rice. Add vegetable broth, onions, or garlic to season them.

As you add grains, remember to keep a large portion of your diet raw by juicing and eating raw vegetables and fruits. Pair your grains (even oatmeal!) with lightly cooked veggies, raw fruits, or a salad.

DAILY FOCUS

"Today I plant the seed."

The truth is that health and happiness take work. And once you arrive at your happy, healthy destination, there is more work to be done to maintain it. So today, focus instead not on whether you gain or lose a pound, whether you feel joyous or blue, or whether or not you love kale, but on the seeds of health and happiness that you are planting. Each little step and each little seed take you farther and farther along your journey. Until one day you wake up and realize health and happiness have been within you all along.

Take five minutes in the morning and evening to sit with your mantra. Recite it, ponder it, and let it flow through you as your motivation for the day.

POSE OF THE DAY

Lie on your stomach with your feet stretched apart at hips distance. Bring your elbows under your shoulders with your forearms parallel. Press your pelvis into the ground, draw your navel up toward your spine to lengthen your lower back, and stretch your chest forward and up. Roll your shoulders back and down to broaden your collarbone as you stretch. Hold for ten breaths.

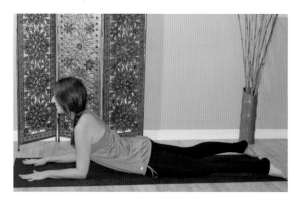

Sphinx

SELF-CARE TIP OF THE DAY

Dry Brushing

Brushing your skin is a fantastic way to remove dead skin cells, increase circulation, and allow more moisture to stay in your skin. Today, grab a coarse bristle brush and start at your toes. In a circular motion, work your way up to you neck, paying extra attention to rough spots like your heels, knees, and elbows. You can lightly dry brush your face if you are comfortable with it.

Try this first thing in the morning, right before you get dressed, or right before you shower.

DAILY ROUTINE

- On your fourth day start by taking a deep breath in and out. Open your eyes and think of three things you are grateful for today.
- Get up and get going. Brush your teeth and scrape your tongue using a metal tongue scraper. This will help you remove unwanted bacteria from your tongue, leave your breath a little fresher, and start to stimulate digestion. All of which will help you feel more bright and shiny today, instead of feeling funky and cranky.
- Head to the kitchen and make some warm water with lemon juice. Drink this first to wake up your digestive system and energize you as you start the day.

- Next, head to your meditation station. Set a timer for five minutes. In your meditation, sit and silently repeat your daily motto. At the end of the five minutes, try your breath and pose of the day. If there is time, give your self-care tip a try and practice your exercise of the day.
- Go ahead and start your daily routine. Make some juice for your first meal. If you are feeling extra famished, light-headed, or even a bit weak, make a smoothie instead or pair your juice with an avocado half or pureed carrots and dates. You might even want to try some steamed or sautéed veggies as part of your breakfast or morning snack today. Asparagus, kale, and spinach all make delicious, flavorful, and detoxifying green morning additions.
- For a mid-morning snack, have a piece of raw fruit or vegetable. The other avocado half also works well in the morning.
- Have lunch around 12 p.m. If you have cooked vegetables, add in a small raw greens salad with it. These enzymes will help you digest and keep releasing toxins.
- For a mid-afternoon snack, smoothies, juices, fruits, and vegetables all work great for an energy boost.
- *Optional time to exercise if not done in morning.
- For dinner, incorporate more steamed and raw foods, such as a raw salad with soup or steamed vegetables. Try to have dinner between 6 and 7 p.m.
- You can have another raw snack after dinner.
- Drink plenty of water, herbal tea, and hot lemon water throughout the day. This will help to keep your digestive system flowing and your skin glowing.
- Before bed, meditate again and see how the mantra might sit differently with you now. Practice your self-care tip and pose if you haven't already.
- At the end of the night, head to bed and settle in for seven to nine hours of sleep. Before drifting off, tell yourself one thing you are proud of accomplishing on your fourth day.

DAY FIVE: EXPERIMENT WITH BEANS, LEGUMES, AND RAW NUTS

MOTTO OF THE DAY

"I am a human being, not a human doing. Don't equate your self-worth with how well you do things in life. You aren't what you do. If you are what you do, then when you don't . . . you aren't." —Dr. Wayne Dyer

On day five, start adding in some nuts, legumes, and beans. Nuts, seeds, and beans are a huge component to a healthy diet. They are all wonderful sources of vitamins, minerals, protein, and fiber, which help you stay energized and full for longer periods of time. However, they can also be hard to digest due to all of the fiber, causing bloating, cramping, and indigestion. To reduce some of these factors, try soaking your nuts and beans before cooking with them. You can also eat these in a variety of ways. Of course, you can stick to the basics—raw, unsalted nuts—or you can get a little creative and start adding nuts to smoothies, desserts, and snacks. Try almond butter instead of traditional peanut butter. Soak a few raw cashews or almonds to add to your favorite smoothie. You'll feel indulgent while still keeping things healthy. After all, you deserve to have a little fun!

And remember to add them in slowly to your diet. As you add in more and more healthy, whole foods, remember to keep eating plenty of fresh greens, vegetables, and fruits. These remain the staple of your diet as the weeks move on and the cleanse turns into a lifestyle.

DAILY FOCUS

"I am not perfect. But I am perfectly me."

The first week of a detox can bring up a multitude of uncertainties and self-doubt. And we can get wrapped up in "doing it right." But when we get into the mindset of all or none, we often lose the connection to the self. We lose the connection to "me." Today, take a few moments to think about what you are beyond your work, your detox, you task list. Know that a few slip-ups along the way are OK. It's trying our best and being OK where we end up that really matters. Remember, perfection often breeds more stress. So let it go, breathe, and relax a bit.

POSE OF THE DAY

During the first week of your detox, you might feel as if you are going through the motions or not quite doing everything right. You might start asking yourself questions like "how can I do this?"; "what if I don't succeed?"; "what happens next?" All of these questions can start to show up in your body as stress and tension. Your movement and breathing practice today will focus on releasing tension through the neck and shoulders, as well as creating a little space between the ears.

Stand with your feet hip distance apart. Reach your arms overhead and clasp your hands. Release your index fingers so they point straight up at the ceiling. Lengthen your arms by your biceps, but drop your shoulders away from your ears. Inhale and lift your chest slightly. Exhale as you lean to the right. Inhale back to the center and exhale as you lean to the left. Continue this for ten rounds. With each breath, feel a little more space between the shoulders and ears and a little less chatter between the ears.

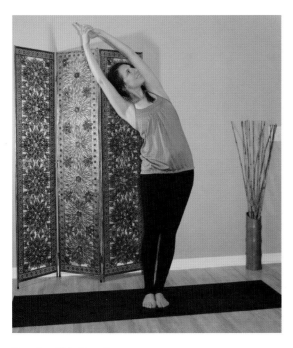 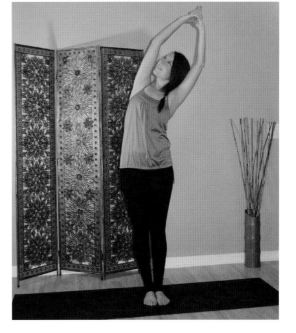

Standing Side Stretch

SELF-CARE TIP OF THE DAY

Warm Bath with Epsom Salts and Sesame Oil

Today, draw a bath. You can make it as warm as you can tolerate. As it fills, add in ½ cup of Epsom salts and two tablespoons of sesame oil. The salt will help to alleviate any muscle tension or soreness and the oil will help to moisturize and warm your skin. You can also add a few drops of lavender essential oil for even more relaxing benefits. Soak in the bath for at least twenty minutes.

DAILY ROUTINE:

- On your fifth day start by taking a deep breath in and out. Open your eyes and think of three things you are grateful for today.
- Get up and get going. Brush your teeth and scrape your tongue using a metal tongue scraper. This will help you remove unwanted bacteria from your tongue, leave your breath a little fresher, and start to stimulate digestion. All of which will help you feel more bright and shiny today, instead of feeling funky and cranky.
- Head to the kitchen and make some warm water with lemon juice. Drink this first to wake up your digestive system and energize you as you start the day.
- Next, head to your meditation station. Set a timer for five minutes. In your meditation, sit and silently repeat your daily motto. At the end of the five minutes, try your breath and pose of the day. If there is time, give your self-care tip a try and practice your exercise of the day.
- Go ahead and start your daily routine. Make some juice for your first meal. If you need something else with it, try some fruits, veggies, oatmeal, or even a handful of raw nuts.
- For a mid-morning snack, have a piece of raw fruit or vegetable or a few nuts.
- Have lunch around 12 p.m. Remember to start adding in the variety slowly, keeping your focus on some raw veggies.
- For a mid-afternoon snack, smoothies, juices, fruits, and vegetables all work great for an energy boost.
- *Optional time to exercise if not done in morning.
- For dinner, again incorporate more of your variety but stick to mostly vegetables and fruits. If most of the meal is cooked, have a handful of greens with your meal. Try to have dinner between 6 and 7 p.m.
- You can have another raw snack after dinner.
- Drink plenty of water, herbal tea, and hot lemon water throughout the day. This will help to keep your digestive system flowing and your skin glowing.
- Before bed, meditate again and see how the mantra might sit differently with you now. Practice your self-care tip and pose if you haven't already.
- At the end of the night, head to bed and settle in for seven to nine hours of sleep. Before drifting off, tell yourself one thing you are proud of accomplishing on your fifth day.

DAY SIX: WHOLE FOODS, WHOLE HEALTH, WHOLE LIFE

MOTTO OF THE DAY

"I have chosen to be happy because it is good for my health." —Voltaire

On day six, you are able to eat a wide variety of whole, healthy foods. Rather than adding in another food group today, take the time to enjoy the foods you have been eating for the past five days. Start to notice how your body feels when you are eating healthy foods. You may notice your digestion has improved, or maybe you are still working out some of the built-up gunk that has been hiding in your system over recent weeks, months, and even years. After each meal, start to pay attention to your energy levels. Notice if you feel tired, energized, hungry, or satisfied, and make note of which foods seem to help you feel your best after eating. When you feel your best, you are able to accomplish more, feel happier, and stay healthier.

Today you get to add one more group to your diet. In addition to veggies, fruits, grains, nuts, and seeds, you can now also start eating beans and legumes. Chickpeas, black beans, and white beans are on the top of the list here. Add them to your meals in a zesty taco bowl or top your salad off with a serving of chickpeas. They are full of fiber, protein, and iron to help you stay energized and strong. Keep eating plenty of vegetables; just think of this as even more variety for you to choose from.

DAILY FOCUS

"I have chosen to be happy, healthy, and free."

It's a big statement, and it's asking a lot, but the more you say it, the more you will begin to believe it. In your journey through your first week, you have focused mainly on food, but it's all in an effort to find the happiness and health that is buried within you. The more you begin to believe you are happy and healthy, the more you will start to make the connection between health, happiness, and caring for your body.

Take five minutes in the morning and evening to sit with your mantra. Recite it, ponder it, and let it flow through you as your motivation for the day.

POSE OF THE DAY

With all of the healthy foods and fiber you've added into your diet, you may notice you feel a little bloated. No worries, this is absolutely normal. To help relieve some bloating and help keep your digestive system running smoothly, you'll focus on gentle folds and twists today.

Lie on your back on a mat. Hug your right knee into your chest. Wrap your arms around your right shin and draw it in closer to you, up and in toward your shoulder. Let your left leg lengthen all the way onto the mat. Hold here for five breaths. Then cross your right leg over your body to the left, into a twist. Hold here for five breaths. Repeat on the opposite side, starting with drawing the left leg into the chest.

SELF-CARE TIP OF THE DAY

Oil Your Skin before You Shower

Before you hop into your shower or bath today, rub oil onto your skin. You can use sesame to help warm your skin if you are feeling cold or dry and coconut oil if your skin feels irritated. Place a liberal amount into your hands and rub it on your arms, legs, and torso and even on your face.

When you get into the shower, the water will be able to cleanse your skin, but the oil will help to lock in moisture, leaving your skin smooth, supple, and healthy.

*Tip: You can use regular coconut oil from your pantry. For the sesame oil, head to the skin-care section of your health food store, rather than the food section. If you use the regular sesame oil, it might smell pretty strong.

DAILY ROUTINE

- On your sixth day start by taking a deep breath in and out. Open your eyes and think of three things you are grateful for today.
- Get up and get going. Brush your teeth and scrape your tongue using a metal tongue scraper. This will

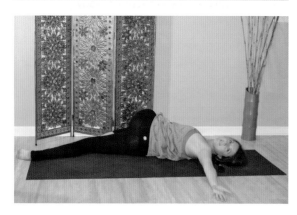

Reclined Single Leg Twist

help you remove unwanted bacteria from your tongue, leave your breath a little fresher, and start to stimulate digestion. All of which will help you feel more bright and shiny today, instead of feeling funky and cranky.

- Head to the kitchen and make some warm water with lemon juice. Drink this first to wake up your digestive system and energize you as you start the day.
- Next head to your meditation station. Set a timer for five minutes. In your meditation, sit and silently repeat your daily motto. At the end of the five minutes, try your breath and pose of the day. If there is time, give your self-care tip a try and practice your exercise of the day.
- Go ahead and start your daily routine. Make some juice for your first meal. As always, you can have some healthy grains, nuts, or extra produce with it.
- For a mid-morning snack, have a piece of raw fruit or vegetable.
- Have lunch around 12 p.m. If you have cooked vegetables and grains, add in a small raw greens salad with it. These enzymes will help you digest and keep releasing toxins.
- For a mid-afternoon snack, smoothies, juices, fruits, and vegetables all work great for an energy boost.
- *Optional time to exercise if not done in morning.
- For dinner, incorporate more steamed and raw produce, such as a raw salad with soup or steamed vegetables, beans, grains, or nuts. Try to have dinner between 6 and 7 p.m.
- You can have another small snack after dinner.
- Drink plenty of water, herbal tea, and hot lemon water throughout the day. This will help to keep your digestive system flowing and your skin glowing.
- Before bed, meditate again and see how the mantra might sit differently with you now. Practice your self-care tip and pose if you haven't already.
- At the end of the night, head to bed and settle in for seven to nine hours of sleep. Before drifting off, tell yourself one thing you are proud of accomplishing on your sixth day.

DAY SEVEN: ESTABLISH NEW HABITS

MOTTO OF THE DAY

"My body is always working toward optimum health."
—Louise Hay

The first week is officially over after day seven. Today take a few moments to soak in the *huge* amount of change you've made in just one week. This week, you've cleaned up your diet, added in more healthy, whole, energizing foods and healthy body practices into your life. After this day, you get to start exercising more and shift your focus away from the food and on to moving your body even more. As you branch out and add more and more into your life, remember that you are now beginning to become firmly established in these healthy roots. By the end of this week and into the beginning of Week 2, allow healthy eating to start to become automatic. As the weeks progress, stick with the food principles that you have learned over this week - eat whole foods, plenty of vegetables, and limit the processed foods. Experiment more with your ingredients, keeping them fresh, whole, and minimally processed. And above all, remember to have fun on your journey back to health. Play around with recipes and find foods that you truly enjoy eating and keep the detoxification process moving along!

Today, find a few of your favorite recipes from the week and make them as a celebration for yourself. No matter how "well" you did this week, know that there is no right or wrong. However far you've come, you have made huge changes and leaps toward living a happier, healthier life.

DAILY FOCUS

"I have the ability, within me, to bring health back to my body and mind."

You have all of the tools and knowledge you need within you to find a healthy balance within your body and mind. This balance brings not only health, but also happiness and peace to you. Sit today with your mantra and notice the ego, or the negative voice, that might speak up to tell you that you can't do this, you don't want to do this, and this whole process is ridiculous. Then let that ego go and know that buried underneath it, you have everything you need to find your health and happiness.

Take 5 minutes in the morning and evening to sit with your mantra. Recite it, ponder it, and let it flow through you as your motivation for the day.

POSE OF THE DAY

As you end the first week, you'll start to wind up your exercise routine. Today, in the last day of the first week, take a few moments to connect to how you are feeling physically.

Start standing with your feet together. Step your left foot back about 2 to 3 feet with all 10 toes facing forward. Keep both legs straight and fold forward, hinging at your hips. Try to keep your spine straight as much as possible. You can release your hands to the ground or to a block if your spine rounds. Hold for 5 breaths. Release back to standing and repeat on the opposite side.

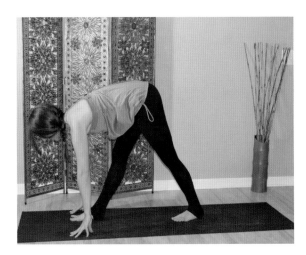

Pyramid

SELF-CARE TIP: DETOX TEA

To help soothe your digestive tract and keep eliminating toxins from your body, make a detoxifying herbal tea. Heat a mug of water until almost boiling. Grate 1 inch of ginger, squeeze one lemon, and scoop a teaspoon of honey. Place them in a French press or tea strainer with you water and brew for 2 minutes. The lemon and ginger will help to soothe and enhance your digestion.

DAILY ROUTINE:

- On your seventh day start by taking 5 deep breaths. With your eyes closed, think of the biggest accomplishment you have made this week.
- Get up and get going. Brush your teeth and scrape your tongue using a metal tongue scraper. This will help you remove unwanted bacteria from your tongue, leave your breath a little fresher, and start to stimulate digestion.
- Head to the kitchen and make some warm water with lemon juice. Drink this first to wake up your digestive system and energize you as you start the day.
- Next head to your meditation station. In your meditation, sit and silently repeat your daily motto. Set a timer for 5 minutes. At the end of the 5 minutes, try your breath and pose of the day. If there

is time, give your self-care tip a try and practice your exercise of the day.

- Go ahead and start your daily routine. Make some juice for your first meal. As always, you can have some healthy grains, nuts, or extra produce with it.
- For a mid-morning snack, have a piece of raw fruit or vegetable.
- Have lunch around 12 p.m. Have fun with it – try a new recipe or a new combination of foods. If you have cooked vegetables and grains, add in a small raw greens salad with it. These enzymes will help you digest and keep releasing toxins.
- For a mid-afternoon snack, smoothies, juices, fruits, and vegetables all work great for an energy boost.
- *Optional time to exercise if not done in AM.
- For dinner, incorporate more steamed and raw produce, such as a raw salad with soup or steamed vegetables, beans, grains, or nuts. Again, celebrate and have fun! Try to have dinner between 6 and 7 pm.
- You can have another small snack after dinner.
- Drink plenty of water, herbal tea, and hot lemon water throughout the day. This will help to keep your digestive system flowing and your skin glowing.
- Before bed, meditate again and see how the mantra might sit differently with you now. Practice your self-care tip and pose if you haven't already.
- At the end of the night, head to bed and settle in for seven to nine hours of sleep. Before drifting off, tell yourself one thing you are proud of accomplishing on your seventh day.

Chapter Seven: Week Two: Restore and Recharge

During week two, the focus shifts from deep cleansing through food, to restoring and recharging with exercise. Since you are still on a cleanse, your exercise should be supportive and energizing, rather than depleting you of energy. You are free to exercise in any way that you like, but you'll find in the back of the book a mapped out exercise plan, which includes more intense exercises starting on week two. These exercises are designed to get your heart rate up, make you sweat, and burn toxins, but also enhance your energy, rather than deplete it.

This week you'll focus on how these exercises improve and support digestion to help you clear out toxins, restore you and release tension, and allow you to sweat a little without becoming completely dehydrated. Anything too intense may cause inflammation and acidity in the body as you try to recover from it, so you'll be exercising, but with a more mindful approach.

As far as your food goes, keep eating whole foods, mostly vegetables and fruits, and add in salads and raw greens. If you have mostly grains or cooked vegetables, pair them with a small salad. Continue to add in more variety and keep each meal interesting and evolving. Play around with your ingredients, keeping about half of each meal raw, with the majority of the meal being vegetables. Have some grains, nuts, beans, and fruit with your veggies. Keep juicing or blending in morning and for snacks throughout the day.

Day Eight

MOTTO OF THE DAY

"Whether you think you can or whether you think you can't, you're right."

—Henry Ford

Today begins your week of adding in more vigorous movement. Stick to your whole foods diet, consuming mostly raw foods, cooked vegetables, and a few whole grains. Keep in mind that your goal here is to feel *more* energized from adding exercise, rather than exhausted.

Getting up and out and moving your body more helps to continue all the cleansing action that you started last week. Now that you have been eating a healthy, clean diet for a week, you are ready to add in more intense exercise to enhance the benefits of the detox. As you move your body more, you'll help to engage the organs in your abdomen, flushing and squeezing the toxins out of them. Exercise also helps you sleep better and can actually give you more energy, which what this detox is all about.

DAILY FOCUS

"I can accomplish anything if I believe in it."

Exercise and working out are sometimes put on the back burner, not because you can't do it, but because of fear. Many exercises require you to stretch slightly outside of your comfort zone, which can be a very scary thing. As you start your day, sit with your mantra. Listen to the words as you recite them silently to yourself. Believe that you can do anything. When you let the fear slip away, you start to have fun with your exercise.

Take 5 minutes in the morning and evening to sit with your mantra. Recite it, ponder it, and let it flow through you as your motivation for the day.

POSE OF THE DAY

When you start to move more, it is common for the hips to become tight. This is because the hips are a major mover for most types of exercise, from running to kick boxing, to dancing, to yoga. When your hips tighten up, you often feel the tightness in your back, thighs, and knees, rather than in the hips themselves.

Today, we'll focus on stretching the hips after your workout. To thoroughly stretch the hips you'll want to open into the hip joint and stretch the front of the hip a.k.a. the hip flexor.

Come onto your hands and knees on a yoga mat. Bring your right knee up toward your right wrist. Slide your shin across, almost parallel to your wrists, until your foot is near the left side of your mat. Reach your left leg straight out behind you on the mat.

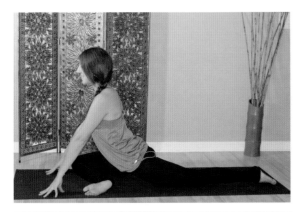

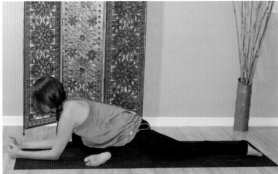

Open Your Hips with Pigeon

Make sure you stay centered over your pelvis and start to lower your chest toward the ground. Hold for 2 to 3 minutes and switch sides. As you open the hips, you cool the body after heating it up during exercise. You also ground some of your energy, which may have become hyper-elevated after your workout.

As you sit in this pose you may feel intense amounts of stretching. Remember to breathe while you stretch and imagine the tension releasing with your exhale.

SELF-CARE TIP: BREATH OF FIRE

Breath of Fire is a strong yogic breath that will help to heat up your body, stoke your digestion, and tone your core. It is also very cleansing for your sinuses, which will help clear out any pressure and fogginess. You do this by pushing your exhale out through your nose and letting your inhale come rushing back in through your nose.

Sit in a cross-legged position or kneeling with a tall spine. Place one hand on your belly. Take a deep breath in. On your exhale, make it short and fast by contracting your abdominal muscles to push the breath out. Keep breathing in and out through your nose for one minute. When you finish take a deep inhale, then exhale through your mouth.

DAILY ROUTINE

- On your eighth day start by taking 2 minutes to reflect on how far you have come in your first week. Reflect on what you have done and what you wish to gain in the next two weeks.
- Get up and get going. Brush your teeth and scrape your tongue using a metal tongue scraper. This will help you remove unwanted bacteria from

your tongue, leave your breath a little fresher, and start to stimulate digestion.

- Head to the kitchen and make some warm water with lemon juice. Drink this first to wake up your digestive system and energize you as you start the day.

- Next head to your meditation station. In your meditation, sit and silently repeat your daily motto. Set a timer for 5 minutes. At the end of the 5 minutes, try your breath and pose of the day. If there is time, give your self-care tip a try and practice your exercise of the day.

- Go ahead and start your daily routine. Make some juice for your first meal. As always, you can have some healthy grains, nuts, or extra produce with it.

- For a mid-morning snack, have a piece of raw fruit or vegetable.

- Have lunch around 12 pm. Have fun with it—try a new recipe or a new combination of foods. If you have cooked vegetables and grains, add in a small raw greens salad with it. These enzymes will help you digest and keep releasing toxins.

- For a mid-afternoon snack, smoothies, juices, fruits, and vegetables all work great for an energy boost.

- *Optional time to exercise if not done in AM.

- For dinner, incorporate more steamed and raw produce, such as a raw salad with soup or steamed vegetables, beans, grains, or nuts. Again, celebrate and have fun! Try to have dinner between 6 and 7 pm.

- You can have another small snack after dinner.

- Drink plenty of water, herbal tea, and hot lemon water throughout the day. This will help to keep your digestive system flowing and your skin glowing.

- Before bed, meditate again and see how the mantra might sit differently with you now. Practice your self-care tip and pose if you haven't already.

- At the end of the night, head to bed and settle in for seven to nine hours of sleep.

Day Nine

MOTTO OF THE DAY

"Strength does not come from physical capacity. It comes from indomitable will."

—Mahatma Gandhi

Today you'll connect to your core—the power center of your body. You core is the center of your body and the connection hub of every piece of your body. Your fingertips, toes, and head all connect back to your center on some level. The fingers connect to the arms, which connect to the shoulders, down into the sides of the ribcage, into the waist, and right into your core. Every move you make comes from the power of your core. When you connect on a deeper level during your workout, you increase not only the core strength, but also the awareness of how your body truly connects. And you also develop the inner core strength of willpower.

DAILY FOCUS

"I have the willpower and strength within me to tap into my core potential."

As you work through your cleanse, there'll be days when you wish to give up and call it quits. But remember, you have the strength and power within you to achieve anything you set your mind to. So set you mind and your vision on becoming the healthiest, happiest version of you possible, right down to your core being.

Take 5 minutes in the morning and evening to sit with your mantra. Recite it, ponder it, and let it flow through you as your motivation for the day.

POSE OF THE DAY

*You'll need a small exercise ball or rolled up pillow/mat to support your back.

Sit on your mat with the soles of your feet on the ground and the ball behind your back. Start with your back straight. Slowly round your spine, pressing your lower back into the ball for support. As you do this, tuck your chin in to your chest and draw your belly

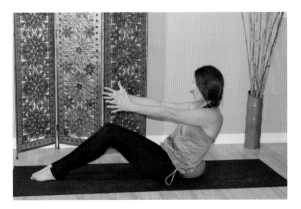

Core Scoop

button into your spine. Keep your knees together. Bring your hands to the back of your legs. Slowly press back into the ball, just an inch or so, and lift back up. Repeat this 12 times, keeping your spine rounded the entire time.

After the 12th time, reach your arms forward. Lean into the ball and hold here. Engage your core. Sweep the right arm back as you twist to the right. Come back to the center and twist the left arm back. Inhale each time you return to the center and exhale each time your twist. Go for 5 on each side.

When you are finished the fifth round, take a few stretches into the hamstrings and hips. These will help stretch the legs, back, and hips, but also cool and calm you after your workout.

SELF-CARE TIP: MOISTURIZE WITH OIL AFTER YOUR SHOWER

Your skin is your largest organ, and to keep it healthy and vibrant, you need to treat it well. Using oil as a moisturizer will moisturize your skin deeply, without any added chemicals, since whatever you put on your body soaks into the rest of your organs.

After your bath or shower, grab your coconut or sesame oil that you previously use before your shower. Lightly rub oil over your arms, legs legs, and torso to deeply moisturize your skin. You'll want to keep it light so you don't feel oily, just deeply moisturized.

DAILY ROUTINE

- On your ninth day start by reaching your arms overhead and stretching from finger tips to toes. Roll onto your right side and pause for a moment. Take a deep breath in and slowly roll up and out of bed.

- Get up and get going. Brush your teeth and scrape your tongue using a metal tongue scraper. This will help you remove unwanted bacteria from your tongue, leave your breath a little fresher, and start to stimulate digestion.

- Head to the kitchen and make some warm water with lemon juice. Drink this first to wake up your digestive system and energize you as you start the day.

- Next head to your meditation station. In your meditation, sit and silently repeat your daily motto. Set a timer for 5 minutes. At the end of the 5 minutes, try your breath and pose of the day. If there is time, give your self-care tip a try and practice your exercise of the day.

- Go ahead and start your daily routine. Make some juice for your first meal. As always, you can have some healthy grains, nuts, or extra produce with it.

- For a mid-morning snack, have a piece of raw fruit or vegetable.

- Have lunch around 12 pm. Have fun with it—try a new recipe or a new combination of foods. If you have cooked vegetables and grains, add in a small raw greens salad with it. These enzymes will help you digest and keep releasing toxins.

- For a mid-afternoon snack, smoothies, juices, fruits, and vegetables all work great for an energy boost.
- *Optional time to exercise if not done in AM.
- For dinner, incorporate more steamed and raw produce, such as a raw salad with soup or steamed vegetables, beans, grains, or nuts. Again, celebrate and have fun! Try to have dinner between 6 and 7 pm.

- You can have another small snack after dinner.
- Drink plenty of water, herbal tea, and hot lemon water throughout the day. This will help to keep your digestive system flowing and your skin glowing.
- Before bed, meditate again and see how the mantra might sit differently with you now. Practice your self-care tip and pose if you haven't already.
- At the end of the night, head to bed and settle in for seven to nine hours of sleep. Before drifting off, tell yourself one thing you are proud of accomplishing today.

Day Ten

MOTTO OF THE DAY:

"Don't worry about failures, worry about the chances you miss when you don't even try."

—Jack Canfield

During this cleanse, you are exercising to feel energized. Before you start to exercise today, take a mental note of how you feel energetically. Do the same thing again post exercise. How do you feel? Are you tired? More awake? Feeling energized? Or feeling depleted? If you feel exhausted post-workout, you may be exercising a little too hard, or not fueling up enough pre- and post-workout.

Pay attention today to the differences between your left and right sides. Notice the places that feel open and the places that feel tight. Exercise from a place of non-judgment, just simply observing with each and every pose. And as you continue throughout the week, keep this mindful pattern with you through all your workouts.

DAILY FOCUS

"I will release fear and take chances."

There are times when we limit what we can do, because we believe we can't do it. We fear change, even on the smallest level, and it can make all the difference. As you begin to exercise, you may notice some fear starting to rise. This resistance to change, the fear of change—whether for good or for bad—can often keep us stagnant. Today, take time to connect to how you are feeling and start to release your fears.

Take 5 minutes in the morning and evening to sit with your mantra. Recite it, ponder it, and let it flow through you as your motivation for the day.

POSE OF THE DAY

Bridge Pose will help you to strengthen your legs and back, while opening your chest and heart center to help release your fears and doubts.

Lay flat on your mat. Bend your knees and walk your feet in toward your glutes, until they line up

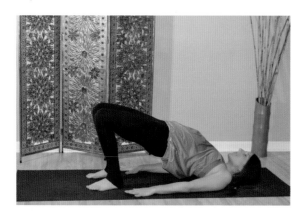

Bridge Pose

directly under your knees. Keep your knees and feet hip distance apart during this pose. Slowly scoop your tailbone off the ground and roll up your spine, pressing your hips up toward the ceiling. Roll your shoulders underneath you and clasp your hands, pushing your clasped fist into the ground. Lift your hips higher, bringing your chest toward your chin. Squeeze your inner thighs for support and engage your abdominal muscles. Hold for 10 breaths and slowly release your hands, arms, shoulders, and then roll down your spine onto your mat. Gently walk you feet to the edges of your mat and knock your knees together to help release your lower back.

SELF-CARE TIP: NETI POT

A Neti Pot is an excellent tool to cleanse your sinuses and clear your head. Neti Pot's gently flush your sinus cavities with a salt water solution to remove any buildup and pressure that might be built up within them.

Neti Pots can be purchased at your local health food store or pharmacy and usually come with salt solution packets. Add your water to the solution in your pot. Tilt your head to the side and open your mouth as you pour the water through your nostril. Switch to the other side when halfway empty.

*Use distilled water only and always clean your Neti Pot.

DAILY ROUTINE

- On your tenth day start by thinking one positive thought or affirmation for your day ahead.
- Get up and get going. Brush your teeth and scrape your tongue using a metal tongue scraper. This will help you remove unwanted bacteria from your tongue, leave your breath a little fresher, and start to stimulate digestion.
- Head to the kitchen and make some warm water with lemon juice. Drink this first to wake up your digestive system and energize you as you start the day.
- Next head to your meditation station. In your meditation, sit and silently repeat your daily motto. Set a timer for 5 minutes. At the end of the 5 minutes, try your breath and pose of the day. If there is time, give your self-care tip a try and practice your exercise of the day.
- Go ahead and start your daily routine. Make some juice for your first meal. As always, you can have some healthy grains, nuts, or extra produce with it.
- For a mid-morning snack, have a piece of raw fruit or vegetable.
- Have lunch around 12 pm. Have fun with it—try a new recipe or a new combination of foods. If you have cooked vegetables and grains, add in a small raw greens salad with it. These enzymes will help you digest and keep releasing toxins.
- For a mid-afternoon snack, smoothies, juices, fruits, and vegetables all work great for an energy boost.
- *Optional time to exercise if not done in AM.
- For dinner, incorporate more steamed and raw produce, such as a raw salad with soup or steamed vegetables, beans, grains, or nuts. Again, celebrate and have fun! Try to have dinner between 6 and 7 pm.
- You can have another small snack after dinner.
- Drink plenty of water, herbal tea, and hot lemon water throughout the day. This will help to keep your digestive system flowing and your skin glowing.
- Before bed, meditate again and see how the mantra might sit differently with you now. Practice your self-care tip and pose if you haven't already.
- At the end of the night, head to bed and settle in for seven to nine hours of sleep.

Day Eleven

MOTTO OF THE DAY

"I can't change the direction of the wind, but I can adjust my sails to always reach my destination."

—Jimmy Dean

Today you'll keep moving, and you'll also add in some supported foods and stretches to help you stay balanced. As you start to exercise more regularly, you may notice your energy needs have shifted and you are a bit hungrier. Today, add a little more intensity to your workout routine and also add in a fresh juice, smoothie, handful of nuts, or energy bar pre- or post-workout. This will help support your body and recharge your energy. You might need more energy before your workout or more energy after your workout to fend off hunger. This is due to the amount of energy you are burning during your workout, but also due to the heat you are building in your body. When your inner heat rises, so can your digestion and hunger rise. To stay balanced and satisfied, try adding in some fresh fruit snacks, juices, or smoothies. And remember to take time to fold, twist, and stretch your hips after your workouts.

DAILY FOCUS

"Whatever my day brings, I have the strength and ability within me to face it."

As you sit in your meditation today, allow yourself to open to the strength within you to face your fears and problems. Let any negativity that has been coming up throughout the weeks to be recognized, acknowledged, and released. You have the strength and ability within you to let them go.

Take 5 minutes in the morning and evening to sit with your mantra. Recite it, ponder it, and let it flow through you as your motivation for the day.

POSE OF THE DAY

Even with a lengthy stretching session or a regular yoga routine, there are times when it feels better to simply sit in the stretch and hold it for a few minutes.

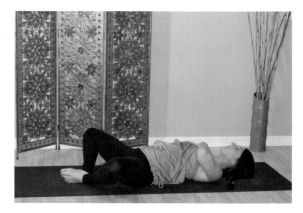

Reclined Cobbler's Pose

After adding in more and more activity to your routine, this pose will help you open into the hips but also help to slow down your breath, cool down, and find relaxation.

Lie flat on your back with the soles of your feet together and your knees open out to the sides. Bring one hand to your belly and one hand to your chest. Simply hold for about 5 minutes, allowing your knees to slowly sink further and further toward the ground. Let gravity do the work here rather than forcing the knees down.

While you rest in the pose, feel the breath flowing in and out beneath your hands. Feel the hands rise on the inhale and fall on the exhale.

SELF-CARE TIP: NECK ROLLER

Grab a foam pool noodle or roll up a bath towel. Lay flat on the ground, your yoga mat, or even your bed. Place the roller underneath your neck and keep it there for about 5 minutes. If you any tension in your neck or shoulders, it might feel intense. If it feels like it is tense, but releasing, stay for a little longer. If it feels too intense, unroll your towel a bit to decrease the intensity of the stretch. As you release, tension and stress that gets built up in your neck and shoulders will be released and removed from your body, creating less stress and tension in your body, mind, and spirit.

DAILY ROUTINE

- On your eleventh day start by rubbing your hands together briskly. Place your palms over your eyes and let the warmth gently wake you.

- Get up and get going. Brush your teeth and scrape your tongue using a metal tongue scraper. This will help you remove unwanted bacteria from your tongue, leave your breath a little fresher, and start to stimulate digestion.

- Head to the kitchen and make some warm water with lemon juice. Drink this first to wake up your digestive system and energize you as you start the day.

- Next head to your meditation station. In your meditation, sit and silently repeat your daily motto. Set a timer for 5 minutes. At the end of the 5 minutes, try your breath and pose of the day. If there is time, give your self-care tip a try and practice your exercise of the day.

- Go ahead and start your daily routine. Make some juice for your first meal. As always, you can have some healthy grains, nuts, or extra produce with it.

- For a mid-morning snack, have a piece of raw fruit or vegetable.

- Have lunch around 12 pm. Have fun with it—try a new recipe or a new combination of foods. If you have cooked vegetables and grains, add in a small raw greens salad with it. These enzymes will help you digest and keep releasing toxins.

- For a mid-afternoon snack, smoothies, juices, fruits, and vegetables all work great for an energy boost.
- *Optional time to exercise if not done in AM.
- For dinner, incorporate more steamed and raw produce, such as a raw salad with soup or steamed vegetables, beans, grains, or nuts. Again, celebrate and have fun! Try to have dinner between 6 and 7 pm.

- You can have another small snack after dinner.
- Drink plenty of water, herbal tea, and hot lemon water throughout the day. This will help to keep your digestive system flowing and your skin glowing.
- Before bed, meditate again and see how the mantra might sit differently with you now. Practice your self-care tip and pose if you haven't already.
- At the end of the night, head to bed and settle in for seven to nine hours of sleep.

Day Twelve

MOTTO OF THE DAY

"You are only one workout away from a good mood."

As movement becomes a part of your daily routine, notice the difference it makes not only in your body's appearance, but in your stress levels, your mind, and in your digestion. Noticing the additional benefits, beyond the purely physical, can help to keep you moving, exercising, and healthy for the long run.

Today use your exercise as a way of de-stressing and finding some clarity. When you exercise, you are not only doing great things physically for your body, but you are doing great things on a more subtle level. Exercise helps to tone the organs, which helps to aid in better digestion. The better your digestion, the less toxic buildup you have, the less bloat you feel, and the better your overall health.

Exercise, when it's not too intense, also helps regulate your blood pressure - that thing that goes up when you are stressed. When your blood pressure lowers, your body recognizes it as a signal to stop stressing and start relaxing.

It also gives you that brief moment in time when there is nothing else to focus on except how your body is moving and grooving. This lets you drop the worries, drop the to-do list making, and simply clear your mind. Find a little extra peace of mind in your workout routine today and onward.

DAILY FOCUS

"I exercise to be the happiest me I can be - physically, emotionally and mentally."

The is no way around it. Exercise can lift your mood, release happy endorphins, and help you focus on something other than the things that are going wrong for you. Take a few minutes to reaffirm this with yourself. The more you hear it, the more you start to believe it. And the more you start to really come to trust and lean on the power of moving your body

Take 5 minutes in the morning and evening to sit with your mantra. Recite it, ponder it, and let it flow through you as your motivation for the day.

POSE OF THE DAY

This stretch work deep into the hips and the back of your leg to help release toxins, built-up energy, and stress, leaving you a little more refreshed and limber post-stretch.

Sit with a tall spine and you legs extended out in front of you. Bring your right ankle across your left thigh, right above your knee. Let your right knee open to the side, so your legs look like a number 4. Keep both feet flexed. Gently press your right knee down to stretch your right hip and fold forward over your legs, grabbing the left foot if accessible. If you can't quite reach your toes or foot, simply rest your hands alongside your shin. Hold for 10 breaths and switch sides.

*If needed, you can do this sitting against a wall to help keep your spine long.

SELF-CARE TIP: COOL TOWEL FOR YOUR EYES

A cool towel placed over your eyes can help you de-stress and recharge almost instantly. Soak a

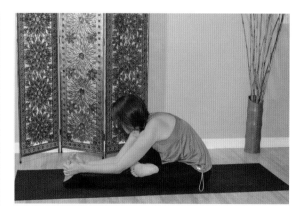

Figure 4 Stretch

towel in water with a few drops each of lavender and eucalyptus essential oils. Place in the refrigerator for at least an hour. Gently place over your eyes while lying down. Stay there for 5 minutes.

DAILY ROUTINE

- On your twelfth day start by taking a deep inhale and exhale. Slowly open your eyes and stretch your arms overhead. Roll onto your side and slowly sit up. Close your eyes again and sit tall, taking three more deep breaths. Check in with your thoughts, your body, and your energy.

- Get up and get going. Brush your teeth and scrape your tongue using a metal tongue scraper. This will help you remove unwanted bacteria from your tongue, leave your breath a little fresher, and start to stimulate digestion.

- Head to the kitchen and make some warm water with lemon juice. Drink this first to wake up your digestive system and energize you as you start the day.

- Next head to your meditation station. In your meditation, sit and silently repeat your daily motto. Set a timer for 5 minutes. At the end of the 5 minutes, try your breath and pose of the day. If there is time, give your self-care tip a try and practice your exercise of the day.

- Go ahead and start your daily routine. Make some juice for your first meal. As always, you can have some healthy grains, nuts, or extra produce with it.

- For a mid-morning snack, have a piece of raw fruit or vegetable.

- Have lunch around 12 pm. Have fun with it—try a new recipe or a new combination of foods. If you have cooked vegetables and grains, add in a small raw greens salad with it. These enzymes will help you digest and keep releasing toxins.

- For a mid-afternoon snack, smoothies, juices, fruits, and vegetables all work great for an energy boost.

- *Optional time to exercise if not done in AM.

- For dinner, incorporate more steamed and raw produce, such as a raw salad with soup or steamed vegetables, beans, grains, or nuts. Again, celebrate and have fun! Try to have dinner between 6 and 7 pm.

- You can have another small snack after dinner.

- Drink plenty of water, herbal tea, and hot lemon water throughout the day. This will help to keep your digestive system flowing and your skin glowing.

- Before bed, meditate again and see how the mantra might sit differently with you now. Practice your self-care tip and pose if you haven't already.

- At the end of the night, head to bed and settle in for seven to nine hours of sleep. If you feel restless before bed, take a moment to breathe deeply and stretch.

Day Thirteen

MOTTO OF THE DAY:

"You live longer once you realize that any time spent being unhappy is wasted."

—Ruth E. Renkl

Today choose your favorite type of exercise and have fun working out!

Whether it's running, yoga, Pilates, or softball, choose your favorite type of exercise and spend some time today practicing and playing it. When you start to connect to something that you really enjoy, it becomes less of a chore and more of a treat. The more you enjoy your exercise, the more likely you are to keep doing it. We easily get wrapped up in what we should be doing, how we should be burning the most energy, and how we should be strengthening with specific weight sets, but if we don't enjoy it, it's almost guaranteed to be temporary.

Take time today to find the workout that is enjoyable to you. Take 60 minutes out of your day for this exercise. Stay indoors and run on your treadmill or pop in a DVD. Dance around your house. Go outside and run, Paddle Board, or swim. Whatever it is that makes your heart sing, makes you feel alive, and clears your mind is the right one for you.

Make a promise to yourself to keep exercising for your overall health and for the fun of it. Observe your energy and how amazing it feels to be healthy. When you nurture your body through healthy foods, exercise, and thoughts, you are more likely to form supportive habits for life.

DAILY FOCUS

"Today I will open to happiness within my workout."

Allow yourself the freedom to be happy during your exercise. Stop beating yourself up physically and emotionally. Stop and actually enjoy the breath moving through you, the pumping of your heart beat, and the strength of your body. Drop the judgment, the "should," and simply start enjoying the freedom of moving your body.

Take 5 minutes in the morning and evening to sit with your mantra. Recite it, ponder it, and let it flow through you as your motivation for the day.

POSE OF THE DAY

This pose will help loosen the back of the legs and shoulders, as well as cool you down after any vigorous exercise. Stand with your feet together. Step your left foot back almost as far as you can. Turn your toes slightly out to the side. Bend your right knee over your ankle and press into the heel of your left foot, rooting it down into the ground. Reach your arms behind you

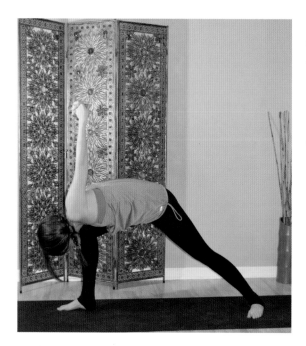

Humble Warrior

and clasp your hands. Stretch your shoulders back as you lift your heart and fold forward, bringing your head toward your right heel. Keep squeezing into your left quadricep to lengthen your leg and plant your left heel down. Hold for 5 breaths and switch sides.

SELF-CARE TIP: MASSAGE

Stress often holds itself in pressure points along our bodies. Today, massage press, or rub these areas of tension in your hands, feet, and shoulders. Squeeze into the center of your hand with your thumb and hold

it for a few seconds. Slowly release and wiggle your fingers. Press your thumbs into the centers of your feet and rub from the balls of your feet to your heels. Reach to your opposite shoulder, at the base of your neck and press your fingertips into your shoulder to release tension. Take a minute to two for each area of tension, slowly starting to let the tension and stress melt away.

DAILY ROUTINE

- On your thirteenth day start by rolling your wrists and ankles and wiggling your fingers and toes to wake up. Slowly open your eyes and stretch your arms overhead. Roll onto your side and slowly sit up. Close your eyes again and sit tall, taking three more deep breaths. Check in with your thoughts, your body, and your energy.

- Get up and get going. Brush your teeth and scrape your tongue using a metal tongue scraper. This will help you remove unwanted bacteria from your tongue, leave your breath a little fresher, and start to stimulate digestion.

- Head to the kitchen and make some warm water with lemon juice. Drink this first to wake up your digestive system and energize you as you start the day.

- Next head to your meditation station. In your meditation, sit and silently repeat your daily motto. Set a timer for 5 minutes. At the end of the

5 minutes, try your breath and pose of the day. If there is time, give your self-care tip a try and practice your exercise of the day.

- Go ahead and start your daily routine. Make some juice for your first meal. As always, you can have some healthy grains, nuts, or extra produce with it.
- For a mid-morning snack, have a piece of raw fruit or vegetable.
- Have lunch around 12 pm. Have fun with it—try a new recipe or a new combination of foods. If you have cooked vegetables and grains, add in a small raw greens salad with it. These enzymes will help you digest and keep releasing toxins.
- For a mid-afternoon snack, smoothies, juices, fruits, and vegetables all work great for an energy boost.
- *Optional time to exercise if not done in AM.

- For dinner, incorporate more steamed and raw produce, such as a raw salad with soup or steamed vegetables, beans, grains, or nuts. Again, celebrate and have fun! Try to have dinner between 6 and 7 pm.
- You can have another small snack after dinner.
- Drink plenty of water, herbal tea, and hot lemon water throughout the day. This will help to keep your digestive system flowing and your skin glowing.
- Before bed, meditate again and see how the mantra might sit differently with you now. Practice your self-care tip and pose if you haven't already.
- At the end of the night, head to bed and settle in for seven to nine hours of sleep. If you feel restless or sore before bed, take a moment to breathe deeply and practice your pose of the day again.

Day Fourteen

MOTTO OF THE DAY

"Clear your mind of can't."

—Samuel Johnson

Today start to see the progress you have made. As you move into the third week of your cleanse, eating and exercising have started to become a regular part of your day, as if they are almost automatic, without even having to think about them. In your third week, try to keep this mindset while you incorporate your new habits into your daily life.

At the end of your second week, you have had time to integrate not only healthy foods into your lifestyle, but also healthy exercise. Notice how it seems just a little easier to fit all of this into your day. It has started to become a habit, part of your lifestyle. You are beginning to put together the pieces of the puzzle that makes up the healthiest, happiest version of you. Today, continue to eat healthy, whole foods and work out to gain energy, have fun, and improve your mood.

DAILY FOCUS

"I simply can. I know I can."

When you let go of "can't", you simply replace it with can. At the end of this second week, you may be feeling a lot of "can't," popping up. As in "I can't continue for another week." In you meditation practice today, sit with the word "can." Start to believe that you really can—you can do or be anything. And you can finish this cleanse with commitment and strength.

Take 5 minutes in the morning and evening to sit with your mantra. Recite it, ponder it, and let it flow through you as your motivation for the day.

POSE OF THE DAY

Ground yourself in your strength.

In a Warrior Pose, you are building strength, opening the hips, and starting to ground into your feet. This grounding of your energy helps to keep you focused and calm.

Stand with your feet apart wider than your hips (about 3 to 4 feet). Turn your right toes to the side and bend your right knee over your ankle. Bring your arms to a "T" and set your gaze steady over your right hand.

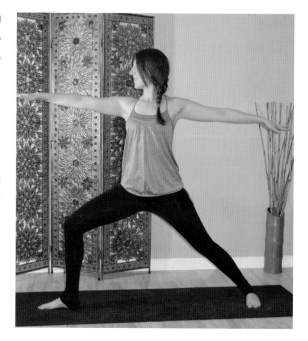
Warrior II

Feel your right big toe press into the ground and the center of your left heel press down. Hold for 5 breaths and switch sides.

SELF-CARE TIP: NON-STOP JOURNALING

Today, for 5 to 10 minutes, journal without stopping. You can start by writing about anything that has been a recurring theme with your thoughts over the past few weeks, you could write about how you have felt over the cleanse, or just start writing and see what comes out. Set a timer and keep writing the entire time. When you can't think of anything else to write about, it's ok, just keep your pen moving, write down "I'm not sure what to say" or anything else that is on your mind at that time. Afterward, you'll have created a little more space in your mind and thoughts, as well as possibly gained some insights into your thought patterns, progress, or anything else that may have been sticking with you throughout the 14 days so far.

DAILY ROUTINE

- On your fourteenth day start by taking a moment to acknowledge the great work you have done over the past few weeks and the strength you have within you.
- Get up and get going. Brush your teeth and scrape your tongue using a metal tongue scraper. This will help you remove unwanted bacteria from your tongue, leave your breath a little fresher, and start to stimulate digestion.
- Head to the kitchen and make some warm water with lemon juice. Drink this first to wake up your digestive system and energize you as you start the day.
- Next head to your meditation station. In your meditation, sit and silently repeat your daily motto. Set a timer for 5 minutes. At the end of the 5 minutes, try your breath and pose of the day. If there is time, give your self-care tip a try and practice your exercise of the day.

- Go ahead and start your daily routine. Make some juice for your first meal. As always, you can have some healthy grains, nuts, or extra produce with it.
- For a mid-morning snack, have a piece of raw fruit or vegetable.
- Have lunch around 12 pm. Have fun with it—try a new recipe or a new combination of foods. If you have cooked vegetables and grains, add in a small raw greens salad with it. These enzymes will help you digest and keep releasing toxins.
- For a mid-afternoon snack, smoothies, juices, fruits, and vegetables all work great for an energy boost.
- *Optional time to exercise if not done in AM.
- For dinner, incorporate more steamed and raw produce, such as a raw salad with soup or steamed vegetables, beans, grains, or nuts. Again, celebrate and have fun! Try to have dinner between 6 and 7 pm.
- You can have another small snack after dinner.
- Drink plenty of water, herbal tea, and hot lemon water throughout the day. This will help to keep your digestive system flowing and your skin glowing.
- Before bed, meditate again and see how the mantra might sit differently with you now. Practice your self-care tip and pose if you haven't already.
- At the end of the night, head to bed and settle in for seven to nine hours of sleep. Before drifting off to sleep, congratulate yourself on finishing your second week.

Chapter Eight: Week Three: Incorporate

Week three is here: You have made it over halfway and are now in the homestretch of your detox program. This means that these habits you are establishing are starting to become part of your everyday routine, and as you embark in this last leg of your journey, you can start to plug them into your "normal" routine so they have a better chance of lasting post-detox.

The focus so far has been mainly on exercise and food, and how they can be used to help you detox and get healthy. As you start to incorporate all of these into your daily routine, let them become almost automatic. The focus shifts now on preparing you for your regular life routines, with the main focus of this week on connecting inward to notice how these changes have started to take root and really change your life. By the end of the week, you'll start to let your focus actually drift away from mapping out exactly what to eat, when to eat, and how much to exercise. Let the pieces fall into place a bit and take notice of all of the knowledge you have learned over the past two weeks.

As this week progresses, start to shift even more out of just the food and fitness portion of your health and start to focus more on your inner happiness and stress levels. Tomorrow, Day Fifteen, you will begin to let go of the restraints of your diet and exercise. Let them come to you naturally, as they are now just a regular part of your routine. Instead, shift your focus to how you feel and how you can settle yourself in moments of negative feelings, or how you can explore and deepen the positive connections. Each day take a few extra minutes to journal or sit and pay attention to how your energy has shifted, how your mood has shifted, and maybe even how your demeanor has shifted. There are so many more positive benefits to a detox than just better looking skin and possibly a smaller waistline. Those are the smaller benefits. The larger benefits are the subtle changes and shifts in your thoughts and your outlook on your life. The key to remember this week is that all of the work you have done so far has led you to this point. By caring for your body through nutritious foods and healthy exercise, you are now able to open to the deeper connection of the inner self. And remember to feel proud of yourself this week! You are nearing the end and have made *HUGE* changes to support the healthy, happy life you deserve.

EXERCISE

This week you will slow down your exercise routine just a bit to get you back into a more normal routine. Remember that the idea is to feel better and more energized after you exercise. Stick to your weekly routine and try to exercise around the same time each day. This way your body will start to crave exercise around that time of day, you will begin to get used to the energizing boost, and you'll start to plan it in as part of your post-detox routine.

FOOD

Try out some new recipes from your book and feel free to make up your own! Make this cleanse as fun as you can by adding in some of your favorite recipes. Just stick to the foods on your do's and don'ts list and get creative.

Use these simple guidelines to help you navigate your menu with ease.

FOOD PRINCIPLES:

- Whole foods
- Cooked and raw
- No gluten
- Limit soy to 2 to 3 times per week
- No dairy; no meat
- Low acid

Day Fifteen

MOTTO OF THE DAY

"There is deep wisdom within our very flesh, if we can only come to our senses and feel it."

—Elizabeth A. Behnke

On day fifteen, take some time to check in on yourself. Start to turn your focus toward how you are feeling on a deeper level, rather than just what you are eating and doing. Are you frustrated, cranky, or upset during this detox? Do you feel restricted? Are you anxious or nervous about the program ending? Or are you feeling more energized, lighter, and overall a little brighter? There is no right or wrong here. Just take a few moments to see how you are feeling. Write it down and see what might be making you feel that way and how you can support it or deepen it.

Focusing all the time on what you are eating, how much you are eating, what type of food, and how and when you exercise can be overwhelming. Hopefully, some of the stress of this is starting to leave you in this third week, as these practices become more a part of your daily life. Even so, today tune in and check in on yourself. Are you feeling stressed or letting the stress start to go? Are you a type A person who feels they need to do a "perfect" cleanse? Are you the type who doesn't give as much effort as you could? Either of these can lead to stress, which ultimately leads to a decrease in health and happiness. Today, and throughout this week, you'll focus on *you* so you can tune in to your inner state.

DAILY FOCUS

"I release my control and allow my senses to guide me. I will listen to my body and my mind in their stillness."

As you let go of the push this week and you let go of the controlled and regimented practices of your cleanse, start to sit in stillness. As you sit, let the control go and let your senses be your guide to open your body and mind. Let the senses be the gateway to the knowledge of how you are doing, feeling, and thriving.

Take 5 minutes in the morning and evening to sit with your mantra. Recite it, ponder it, and let it flow through you as your motivation for the day.

POSE OF THE DAY

Feel your feet and push down into them.

Chair pose is similar to a squat with the legs and feet together. In Chair, you are pushing your energy downward to connect into the earth beneath you. You feel the weight of the body sinking into the hips and pressing through the heels.

Stand with your feet together and your hands together at your heart. Bend your knees and hinge at

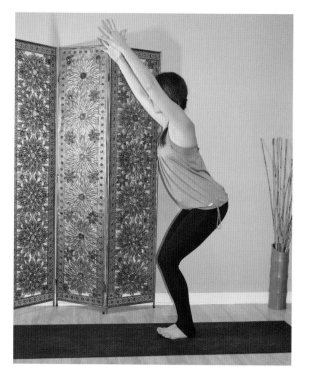

Chair Pose

your hips. Give your toes a little wiggle to feel your heels pressing down. Hold for 10 deep, slow breaths.

SELF-CARE TIP: STEAM FACIAL

Steam can help open pores, clarify your skin, awaken your senses, and relax you.

Warm a large bowl of water until it is hot and steamy, but does not burn you. Sprinkle in a few drops of lavender essential oil to calm you, eucalyptus to open you pores and sinuses, and tea tree oil to cleanse. Place a large towel over your head and lean over the bowl. Let the towel drape completely over it to lock in the steam and moisture. Breathe deeply and stay until the steam disappears.

DAILY ROUTINE:

- On your fifteenth day start by being grateful for taking the time to connect back to you. Scan through your body from your toes and fingertips, up through your limbs, into your torso, up your neck, and into your head. Note any areas that feel tense and any places that feel open. Take a deep breath into them and exhale out though your mouth.
- Get up and get going. Brush your teeth and scrape your tongue using a metal tongue scraper. This will help you remove unwanted bacteria from your tongue, leave your breath a little fresher, and start to stimulate digestion.
- Head to the kitchen and make some warm water with lemon juice. Drink this first to wake up your digestive system and energize you as you start the day.
- Next head to your meditation station. In your meditation, sit and silently repeat your daily motto. Set a timer for 5 minutes. At the end of the 5 minutes, try your breath and pose of the day. If there is time, give your self-care tip a try and practice your exercise of the day.
- Go ahead and start your daily routine. Make some juice for your first meal. As always, you can have some healthy grains, nuts, or extra produce with it.
- For a mid-morning snack, have a piece of raw fruit or vegetable.
- Have lunch around 12 pm. Have fun with it—try a new recipe or a new combination of foods. If you have cooked vegetables and grains, add in a small raw greens salad with it. These enzymes will help you digest and keep releasing toxins.
- For a mid-afternoon snack, smoothies, juices, fruits, and vegetables all work great for an energy boost.
- *Optional time to exercise if not done in AM.
- For dinner, incorporate more steamed and raw produce, such as a raw salad with soup or steamed vegetables, beans, grains, or nuts. Again, celebrate and have fun! Try to have dinner between 6 and 7 pm.

- You can have another small snack after dinner.
- Drink plenty of water, herbal tea, and hot lemon water throughout the day. This will help to keep your digestive system flowing and your skin glowing.

- Before bed, meditate again and see how the mantra might sit differently with you now. Practice your self-care tip and pose if you haven't already.
- At the end of the night, head to bed and settle in for seven to nine hours of sleep.

Day Sixteen

MOTTO OF THE DAY

"The body never lies."

—Martha Graham

On the sixteenth day, start to become more aware of your newfound health and energy. Pay attention to how you feel before and after eating your meals and workouts. Notice any changes or shifts that occur after these activities. Start to think of this as a meditation practice. Observe your body and mind after each meal, snack, or workout. Start to notice if the foods, drinks, and activities are enhancing or depleting your energy levels.

DAILY FOCUS

"I am rooted in life and in myself. I am stable, safe and secure. I love my body and trust in its wisdom."

The more you get grounded in your own body, the more you can start to tune in to the sensations within it. Remember, the body never lies. The sensations, aches, pains, openings, releases you feel within your body are the truth. They are what guide you to establish trust. The mind often interprets these sensations differently than they are. Start to trust your body. Trust what you feel.

Take 5 minutes in the morning and evening to sit with your mantra. Recite it, ponder it, and let it flow through you as your motivation for the day.

POSE OF THE DAY

This standing pose firmly awakens the legs, rooting from the pelvis, down the legs, and into the feet.

Stand with your feet apart three to four feet. Turn your right toes to the side. Reach your arms to a "T" shape, straight out from your shoulders. Push your right hip crease toward your left heel and reach your right fingertips forward. Keep the arms in a "T," but reach the right arm toward your right big toe and the left arm up to the ceiling. The hips will keep pushing back toward the left leg and foot.

Both legs are straight in this pose. Push your left heel firmly into the ground and press just as firmly into your right big toe.

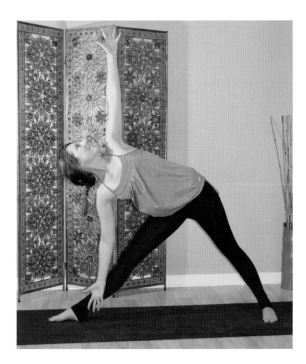

Triangle Pose

- Hold for 10 breaths and switch sides.

SELF-CARE TIP: SOAK UP SOME SUNSHINE!

If it's sunny at all outside, or even if it's cold and dreary, head outside for a walk, a frolic, or just sit outside and have a cup of tea. The sunshine and air outside will help to reinvigorate you, wake you up, and refresh you. Try this early in the morning or anytime during the day that you feel tired or need a break. Feel refreshed and recharged by the sunlight.

DAILY ROUTINE

- On your sixteenth day start by taking a deep breath in and out through your nose. Inhale and feel your belly fill. Exhale to let it go. Repeat this 5 times.
- Get up and get going. Brush your teeth and scrape your tongue using a metal tongue scraper. This will help you remove unwanted bacteria from your tongue, leave your breath a little fresher, and start to stimulate digestion.
- Head to the kitchen and make some warm water with lemon juice. Drink this first to wake up your digestive system and energize you as you start the day.
- Next head to your meditation station. In your meditation, sit and silently repeat your daily motto. Set a timer for 5 minutes. At the end of the 5 minutes, try your breath and pose of the day. If there is time, give your self-care tip a try and practice your exercise of the day.
- Go ahead and start your daily routine. Make some juice for your first meal. As always, you can have some healthy grains, nuts, or extra produce with it.
- For a mid-morning snack, have a piece of raw fruit or vegetable.
- Have lunch around 12 pm. Have fun with it—try a new recipe or a new combination of foods. If you have cooked vegetables and grains, add in a

small raw greens salad with it. These enzymes will help you digest and keep releasing toxins.

- For a mid-afternoon snack, smoothies, juices, fruits, and vegetables all work great for an energy boost.
- *Optional time to exercise if not done in AM.
- For dinner, incorporate more steamed and raw produce, such as a raw salad with soup or steamed vegetables, beans, grains, or nuts. Again, celebrate and have fun! Try to have dinner between 6 and 7 pm.

- You can have another small snack after dinner.
- Drink plenty of water, herbal tea, and hot lemon water throughout the day. This will help to keep your digestive system flowing and your skin glowing.
- Before bed, meditate again and see how the mantra might sit differently with you now. Practice your self-care tip and pose if you haven't already.
- At the end of the night, head to bed and settle in for seven to nine hours of sleep.

Day Seventeen

MOTTO OF THE DAY

"To lose our connection with the body is to become spiritually homeless. Without an anchor, we float aimlessly, battered by the winds and waves of life."

—Anodea Judith

On Day seventeen, you are half way through your last week of the detox. Today is when you can really begin to practice your new habits in your daily routine. Take careful look at how your day has been flowing throughout recent weeks. By now, hopefully, you are able to incorporate healthy eating and exercise into your diet without too much thought or stress. But maybe meditation or moments of stillness might be harder to keep up. Or maybe you know that you are the type of person who strays completely once the structure is over. Start planning now. Make some charts, map it on your calendar, or add reminders to your phone. The more you take charge now, the less stressed you'll be the first day post detox. Start to think about how you can incorporate these into your regular routine, once you don't have the days mapped out for you anymore. Today take a few moments to look at your schedule and see where you can find time to shop, meditate, cook, and exercise once the Detox is over.

Where can you find time to meditate? When can you exercise? What foods will you make a priority? Start now to prepare yourself for the end of the week.

You've got this! You've made it so far already; you have every tool within you to make this happen!

DAILY FOCUS

"My body is my home and I love and respect it."

Within your skin, within your bones, your muscles, your tissues, is where your true home resides. No matter where you live, what you experience, or how you feel, your inner home travels with you, always steady, always loyal. Take a moment today to reaffirm your commitment to treat your home, where your soul resides, with love and respect. Each and every moment of each and every day.

Take 5 minutes in the morning and evening to sit with your mantra. Recite it, ponder it, and let it flow through you as your motivation for the day.

POSE OF THE DAY

Sit on a mat, pillow, cushion, or blanket with your legs stretched out in front of you. Lengthen your spine and slide your right leg open to the edge of your mat. Bring the sole of your left foot to you right inner thigh. Turn over your right leg, keeping your spine long. Slowly hinge at your hips to fold forward. You can rest your hands on the ground, your shin, or reach for your toes. Just keep your chest reaching toward your shin, your gaze at your toes, and your shoulder-blades drawing back and down to help lengthen your spine as you fold. Hold for 10 breaths and switch sides.

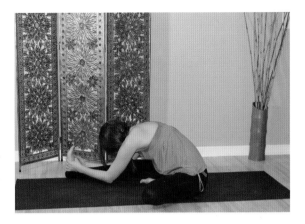

Half Forward Fold

SELF-CARE TIP: MEDITATIVE WALK

Nature has a way of taking us out of our head, into our bodies, and into the world. When we connect to nature, our stress levels tend to come down and we can get into a meditative state of mind more easily than on a treadmill or at the gym.

Today, head outside for a slow, quiet walk somewhere in nature—maybe the woods, a lake, the beach, your neighborhood, or a nearby park, somewhere without a lot of traffic. With each step, feel your heel, arch, and toes press toward the ground. You can count your step or repeat your mantra with each step. The idea is that you start to tune in to the moment and into each step, letting all other worries, aches, stress, and tension drift away. Keep doing this for 5 to 10 minutes, or 100 steps.

DAILY ROUTINE

- On your seventeenth day start by stretching your arms overhead. Reach through your fingertips and toes. Take a deep breath in and as you exhale sit up and reach for your toes.

- Get up and get going. Brush your teeth and scrape your tongue using a metal tongue scraper. This will help you remove unwanted bacteria from your tongue, leave your breath a little fresher, and start to stimulate digestion.

- Head to the kitchen and make some warm water with lemon juice. Drink this first to wake up your digestive system and energize you as you start the day.

- Next head to your meditation station. In your meditation, sit and silently repeat your daily motto. Set a timer for 5 minutes. At the end of the 5 minutes, try your breath and pose of the day. If there is time, give your self-care tip a try and practice your exercise of the day.

- Go ahead and start your daily routine. Make some juice for your first meal. As always, you can have some healthy grains, nuts, or extra produce with it.

- For a mid-morning snack, have a piece of raw fruit or vegetable.

- Have lunch around 12 pm. Have fun with it—try a new recipe or a new combination of foods. If you have cooked vegetables and grains, add in a small raw greens salad with it. These enzymes will help you digest and keep releasing toxins.

- For a mid-afternoon snack, smoothies, juices, fruits, and vegetables all work great for an energy boost.

- *Optional time to exercise if not done in AM.

- For dinner, incorporate more steamed and raw produce, such as a raw salad with soup or steamed vegetables, beans, grains, or nuts. Again, celebrate and have fun! Try to have dinner between 6 and 7 pm.

- You can have another small snack after dinner.

- Drink plenty of water, herbal tea, and hot lemon water throughout the day. This will help to keep your digestive system flowing and your skin glowing.

- Before bed, meditate again and see how the mantra might sit differently with you now. Practice your self-care tip and pose if you haven't already.

- At the end of the night, head to bed and settle in for seven to nine hours of sleep. If your mind is wandering before bed, sit and journal to get all of your thoughts out. Then sink into a forward fold and take three deep breaths.

Day Eighteen

MOTTO OF THE DAY

"Here in this body are the sacred rivers, here are the sun and the moon, as well as the pilgrimage places. I have not encountered another temple as blissful as my own."

—Saraha Doha

You are almost there. Take the time today to have fun with your food and fitness. One of the best ways to stay grounded and ward off stress - treat yourself once in a while. Treating yourself is one of the main focuses on self-care. If you don't take time to treat yourself, you'll find you start to grow grumpy and stressed. Treat yourself to a workout or healthy food you have wanted to try, but maybe have been putting off. Get creative in the kitchen and try a fun new or favorite recipe. And become creative with your workout. Try something new and exciting, or head out for your favorite workout. Maybe take a yoga or barre class at a studio you've been waiting to try. And just have fun! Do you have a healthy food or restaurant you keep finding reasons to put off trying? Go ahead and treat yourself today. You've made it so far, and you only have a few days to go. Treat yourself well today, so you'll be better able to deal with stress tomorrow and beyond.

DAILY FOCUS

"My body is my temple and I will treat it with love."

Your body is your temple. It is the place that holds the you that has no boundaries. Treat yourself with love, stay grounded with that love, and let the rest melt away.

Take 5 minutes in the morning and evening to sit with your mantra. Recite it, ponder it, and let it flow through you as your motivation for the day.

POSE OF THE DAY

This helps your stretch the legs after working out, plus it grounds your energy, keeping you steady and de-stressed.

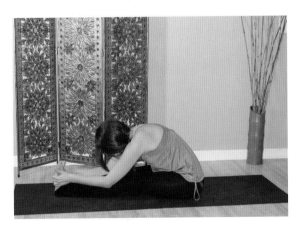

Seated Forward Fold

Sit on a mat, pillow, cushion, or yoga block. Reach your legs straight out in front of you. Feel your spine lengthen as you sit tall. Let the ribcage lift off the waist and draw your shoulder blades back and down. Hinge forward slightly from your hip, keeping your spine long. Think chin to shins as you fold to help you keep length through the spine. Hold for 10 breaths. Note* Your hands do not have to reach your toes, you can always place them on the shins or beside your legs.

SELF-CARE TIP: SLEEP

One of the best and easiest ways to treat yourself is to get extra sleep. Sometimes, no matter how much sleep you get, you might get worn out of just need a quick nap to recharge. This is usually your bodies way of telling you to take a break, heal, and rebuild before you get sick.

Today, take some time, even just 10 minutes, to get a little extra sleep. If you are feeling tired during the day, take a nap. You can also sleep in a few extra minutes or head to bed a few minutes earlier. However you do it, allow yourself these few moments to completely rest, recover, and recharge.

DAILY ROUTINE

- On your eighteenth day start by setting your own intention for the day ahead. What would you like to bring into your life today? How would you like today to feel?

- Get up and get going. Brush your teeth and scrape your tongue using a metal tongue scraper. This will help you remove unwanted bacteria from your tongue, leave your breath a little fresher, and start to stimulate digestion.

- Head to the kitchen and make some warm water with lemon juice. Drink this first to wake up your digestive system and energize you as you start the day.

- Next head to your meditation station. In your meditation, sit and silently repeat your daily motto. Set a timer for 5 minutes. At the end of the 5 minutes, try your breath and pose of the day. If there is time, give your self-care tip a try and practice your exercise of the day.

- Go ahead and start your daily routine. Make some juice for your first meal. As always, you can have some healthy grains, nuts, or extra produce with it.

- For a mid-morning snack, have a piece of raw fruit or vegetable.

- Have lunch around 12 pm. Have fun with it—try a new recipe or a new combination of foods. If you have cooked vegetables and grains, add in a small raw greens salad with it. These enzymes will help you digest and keep releasing toxins.

- For a mid-afternoon snack, smoothies, juices, fruits, and vegetables all work great for an energy boost.

- *Optional time to exercise if not done in AM.
- For dinner, incorporate more steamed and raw produce, such as a raw salad with soup or steamed vegetables, beans, grains, or nuts. Again, celebrate and have fun! Try to have dinner between 6 and 7 pm.
- You can have another small snack after dinner.
- Drink plenty of water, herbal tea, and hot lemon water throughout the day. This will help to keep your digestive system flowing and your skin glowing.
- Before bed, meditate again and see how the mantra might sit differently with you now. Practice your self-care tip and pose if you haven't already.
- At the end of the night, head to bed and settle in for seven to nine hours of sleep. If you feel extra awake when you head to bed, try a cup of warm water or chamomile tea to soothe you into sleep.

Day Nineteen

MOTTO OF THE DAY

"It's not who you are that holds you back, it's who you think you're not."

—Anonymous

Today put your skills to the test in a social setting. Go out to eat with friends or family, or invite people over to your house. In a social setting, see what it's like to continue with your patterns. As you head out for some social engagements, bring your tools with you. Schedule in your exercise and daily tips, poses, and practices.

For your food choices, check where you are going ahead of time. Most places have some kind of vegetarian, gluten free option. If not, make something ahead of time. Since there is no alcohol or coffee on the cleanse, try sparkling water and lime or green tea. Get home in time for plenty of sleep. It sounds restrictive, but when you take care of yourself and stay energized, you are better able to enjoy all of life's experiences.

Remember, it's not about deprivation - enjoy real food, real fun, and real energy!

DAILY FOCUS

"I will not let preconceived notions about who I am hold me back."

We are often too easy to judge ourselves based on who we think we are or are not. Today in your meditation, let go of the images you have of yourself that are limiting. Any notions that you are not enough, that you are not worth it, or that you are not perfectly you can start to fall away. Replace these with the thought "I am enough, I am worth it, and I am perfectly me."

Take 5 minutes in the morning and evening to sit with your mantra. Recite it, ponder it, and let it flow through you as your motivation for the day.

POSE OF THE DAY

This pose helps to ground you by pushing the weight into your feet and supports the cleansing process by wringing toxins from the organs.

Stand with your feet together. Sit into a squat with your knees together. Bring your hand together at your heart. Keep the knees bent and hinge at the hips. Slowly twist to your right, hooking the left upper arm across your right thigh. Make sure your knees stay aligned together. Hold for 5 breaths and switch to the other side.

SELF-CARE TIP: CHEW YOUR FOOD

Since you might be heading out for a meal or dining with family and friends, spend some extra time slowing down and being aware of how you feel while you are eating. It is very common to eat quickly, not fully chewing, tasting, or enjoying our meals. This leads to poor digestion and also can lead to overeating, bloating, and fullness.

Today, take time to really chew your food. Chew each bite 20 times. It might seem like a lot, but you'll probably notice how much more you taste and how your body feels with eat bite. Stay tuned in and aware by chewing slowly and with intention.

DAILY ROUTINE

- On your nineteenth day start by taking a deep inhale and exhale. Remind yourself that you are an amazing being who can do anything you believe in.
- Get up and get going. Brush your teeth and scrape your tongue using a metal tongue scraper. This will help you remove unwanted bacteria from your tongue, leave your breath a little fresher, and start to stimulate digestion.

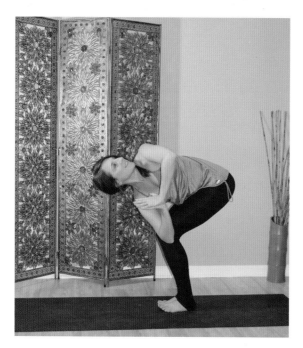

Chair Twist

- Head to the kitchen and make some warm water with lemon juice. Drink this first to wake up your digestive system and energize you as you start the day.
- Next head to your meditation station. In your meditation, sit and silently repeat your daily motto. Set a timer for 5 minutes. At the end of the 5 minutes, try your breath and pose of the day. If there is time, give your self-care tip a try and practice your exercise of the day.
- Go ahead and start your daily routine. Make some juice for your first meal. As always, you can have some healthy grains, nuts, or extra produce with it.
- Have lunch around 12 pm. Have fun with it—try a new recipe or a new combination of foods. If you have cooked vegetables and grains, add in a small raw greens salad with it. These enzymes will help you digest and keep releasing toxins.
- For a mid-afternoon snack, smoothies, juices, fruits, and vegetables all work great for an energy boost.
- *Optional time to exercise if not done in AM.
- For dinner, incorporate more steamed and raw produce, such as a raw salad with soup or steamed vegetables, beans, grains, or nuts. Again, celebrate and have fun! Try to have dinner between 6 and 7 pm.
- You can have another small snack after dinner.
- Drink plenty of water, herbal tea, and hot lemon water throughout the day. This will help to keep your digestive system flowing and your skin glowing.
- Before bed, meditate again and see how the mantra might sit differently with you now. Practice your self-care tip and pose if you haven't already.
- At the end of the night, head to bed and settle in for seven to nine hours of sleep. Plan ahead so you can get your full amount of sleep.

Day Twenty

MOTTO OF THE DAY

"Strive for progress, not perfection"

—Unknown

Take today to simply reflect. Look at how far you have come and how far you can still go with your last two days. By now, you have put in the effort and made big changes not only to your diet and exercise, but to your overall happiness. Reflect on what was the biggest turning point for you. What was your biggest challenge and what was your biggest triumph?

Chances are, you've had many of these along the way. Where did you struggle and what did you find easy? These are both valuable tools for you to use in the final two days and onward post-detox. Look at the triumphs you made and what has been easy for you. These are the things that you can easily incorporate into your daily routines. These are where you can stress less and find some simplification. Where did you struggle and what challenged you? These are the things you can use as you move forward. These are your tools to know where to go next as you have incorporated all of these things into your routine.

Sit today and reflect. Maybe write it down. Hang it up where you can see it or keep it in a journal that you can come back to each day. These will become your goals and your affirmations as you move on.

DAILY FOCUS

"I am not perfect, but I am perfectly me."

Today, take it one step further to drop judgment, find more love, and get grounded in your positive affirmations. When we detox, sometimes we strive for perfection. And in and out of cleanses, we often strive for the perfect life, the perfect diet, the perfect body, and the perfect image. But more often than not, we let go of healthy habits in an effort to find these things. Rather than living up to our own unattainable goals, let's simply accept that we are not perfect. But instead decide that you are perfectly you—just as you are.

Take 5 minutes in the morning and evening to sit with your mantra. Recite it, ponder it, and let it flow through you as your motivation for the day.

POSE OF THE DAY

Find a sense of calm and comfort in this pose, bringing you back to your grounded, true self.

Sit on your heels on a yoga or exercise mat. Open your knees to the edges of our mat and fold forward. Keep your hips to your heels and bring your forehead to the ground. Stretch your arms in front of you. Take a deep breath in for a count of 5 and out for a count of 6. Repeat this 10 times.

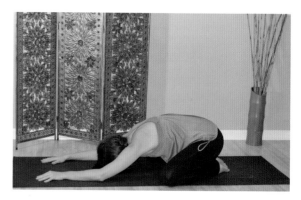

Child's Pose

SELF-CARE TIP: DE-CLUTTER

Clutter in your home and your work space can lead to clutter in your thoughts and stress in your body.

Take some time today to de-clutter your work space, bedroom, kitchen counter, or whatever holds the most clutter for you. Let go of the things that no longer serve you and make space for the things that do.

DAILY ROUTINE

- On your twentieth day slowly open your eyes and roll onto your side. Slowly sit up and open your eyes. Inhale and reach your arms overhead. Clasp your hands and exhale as you lean over to the right. Inhale to lift back up and exhale to lean over to the left. Inhale reach back up and exhale release your hands.

- Get up and get going. Brush your teeth and scrape your tongue using a metal tongue scraper. This will help you remove unwanted bacteria from your tongue, leave your breath a little fresher, and start to stimulate digestion.

- Head to the kitchen and make some warm water with lemon juice. Drink this first to wake up your digestive system and energize you as you start the day.

- Next head to your meditation station. In your meditation, sit and silently repeat your daily motto. Set a timer for 5 minutes. At the end of the 5 minutes, try your breath and pose of the day. If there is time, give your self-care tip a try and practice your exercise of the day.

- Go ahead and start your daily routine. Make some juice for your first meal. As always, you can have some healthy grains, nuts, or extra produce with it.

- For a mid-morning snack, have a piece of raw fruit or vegetable.

- Have lunch around 12 pm. Have fun with it—try a new recipe or a new combination of foods. If you have cooked vegetables and grains, add in a small raw greens salad with it. These enzymes will help you digest and keep releasing toxins.

- For a mid-afternoon snack, smoothies, juices, fruits, and vegetables all work great for an energy boost.

- *Optional time to exercise if not done in AM.

- For dinner, incorporate more steamed and raw produce, such as a raw salad with soup or steamed vegetables, beans, grains, or nuts. Again, celebrate and have fun! Try to have dinner between 6 and 7 pm.

- You can have another small snack after dinner.

- Drink plenty of water, herbal tea, and hot lemon water throughout the day. This will help to keep your digestive system flowing and your skin glowing.

- Before bed, meditate again and see how the mantra might sit differently with you now. Practice your self-care tip and pose if you haven't already.

- At the end of the night, head to bed and settle in for seven to nine hours of sleep. If you feel restless before bed, come back into your child's pose for 1 to 3 minutes.

Day Twenty-One

MOTTO OF THE DAY:

"The finish line is just the beginning of a whole new race."

—Unknown

You made it!

Today is the last day of your cleanse, which means you have spent the last 21 days healing, detoxing, and making a deeper connection with you. This is no small feat. It takes determination, focus, forgiveness, and a sense of humbleness. And you did it. Take today to congratulate yourself and celebrate in some way. Celebrate and plan for your future. Head out. Go shopping. Splurge on a delicious, healthy meal outside of the house or cook yourself something fabulous. Maybe a celebration out with friends or a small celebration with just you or a close loved one. Whatever you decide to do, remember that you are celebrating your health and happiness and all the effort it took to re-find it. You made it three weeks and put in the hard work to become the healthiest and happiest version of you. Celebrate all the gains you have made and all of the tools you have unleashed over the past few weeks. Show your friends and family how amazing you feel and share with them the tools *they* have to become happy and healthy. Spread the word and spread the love. You deserve it!

Congratulations for your work toward that healthy, happy life you deserve.

DAILY FOCUS

"I am healthy, I am happy. I am living the life I deserve."

Even if you don't fully believe it, it is true. The more you recite this mantra, the more you start to feel it. After all of your hard work, and before your hard work even began, it was true. You are healthy. You are happy. You are living the life you deserve.

Take 5 minutes in the morning and evening to sit with your mantra. Recite it, ponder it, and let it flow through you as your motivation for the day.

POSE OF THE DAY

There is no pose more centering, more grounding, more restful than Savasana. In Savasana, try to find complete stillness of your body. Allow that stillness to transfer over into your thoughts.

Simply lie flat on your mat or the ground. Let your legs open and your arms rest a few inches from the body with the palms facing up. Slightly tuck your chin and close your eyes. As you lay here, there is nothing more to do than to simply breathe. Not a strong inhale and exhale. Just simply observe the breath. Feel the body grow heavy, rooting and relaxing into your mat.

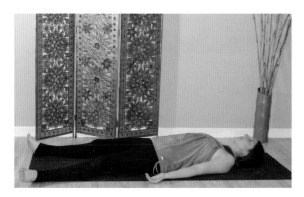
Savasana

And stay here for at least 5 minutes. After five minutes, rollover onto your right side and slowly roll up to a seated position.

SELF-CARE TIP: AROMATHERAPY

Certain scents can trigger you to relax, recharge, or even help you detoxify. Today, grab an essential oil or aromatherapy candle that you found the most useful during the cleanse. If you needed more relaxation, go for lavender. If you needed cleansing, try tea tree oil. If you need to recharge and release, eucalyptus will work. And if you need to awaken and refresh, peppermint oil will help brighten your day. Light your candle or use a diffuser with your oil and have that scent with you while you work, while you take a bath, in your kitchen while you cook, or as you settle down to watch a movie or read a book. Breathe it in and soak it up. You deserve it!

DAILY ROUTINE

- On your twenty-first day start by taking a deep inhale and exhale. You made it. Today is the last day. Let the accomplishment sink in. Breathe it in and congratulate yourself on every moment and every triumph from the past three weeks.

- Get up and get going. Brush your teeth and scrape your tongue using a metal tongue scraper. This will help you remove unwanted bacteria from your tongue, leave your breath a little fresher, and start to stimulate digestion.

- Head to the kitchen and make some warm water with lemon juice. Drink this first to wake up your digestive system and energize you as you start the day.

- Next head to your meditation station. In your meditation, sit and silently repeat your daily motto. Set a timer for 5 minutes. At the end of the 5 minutes, try your breath and pose of the day. If there is time, give your self-care tip a try and practice your exercise of the day.

- Go ahead and start your daily routine. Make some juice for your first meal. As always, you can have some healthy grains, nuts, or extra produce with it.

- For a mid-morning snack, have a piece of raw fruit or vegetable.

- Have lunch around 12 pm. Have fun with it—try a new recipe or a new combination of foods. If you have cooked vegetables and grains, add in a small raw greens salad with it. These enzymes will help you digest and keep releasing toxins.

- For a mid-afternoon snack, smoothies, juices, fruits, and vegetables all work great for an energy boost.
- *Optional time to exercise if not done in AM.
- For dinner, incorporate more steamed and raw produce, such as a raw salad with soup or steamed vegetables, beans, grains, or nuts. Again, celebrate and have fun! Try to have dinner between 6 and 7 pm.
- You can have another small snack after dinner.
- Drink plenty of water, herbal tea, and hot lemon water throughout the day. This will help to keep your digestive system flowing and your skin glowing.
- Before bed, meditate again and see how the mantra might sit differently with you now. Practice your self-care tip and pose if you haven't already.
- At the end of the night, head to bed and settle in for seven to nine hours of sleep. If you feel restless, lay in Savasana for a few minutes, finding that same stillness and restfulness that you worked on earlier.

Chapter Nine: Stepping Out of the Detox

As you complete your 21 day cleanse, there are a few things to keep in mind. After all, this is just the beginning of your new journey. You have learned new concepts, unburied tools, and connected deeper to uncover the healthy, happy you that has been there all along. As you start to move away from the structure of your cleanse, this is your time to take the things you have learned and see how they fit into your everyday experiences.

First, consider where you are now and where you were when you started this program. Along the way you have picked up new tools, discovered strengths within yourself, and made new, healthy lifestyle habits. Even if you had healthy practices beforehand, you have enhanced these in every aspect of your life. When you move out of the detox, keep these practices with you as much as possible. Notice how you feel and think about how you felt at the beginning of your detox. There was a reason that you felt the need to improve your health. Use that reason as your guide into the next phase of your life post-detox.

Second, there is no need to rush. You may find that a few of the daily practices or food choices just aren't practical for you on a daily basis or they may not fit into your budget in the long-term. Stick to the habits that come the most naturally to you now and use the others when you can. Find the things that keep you feeling healthy and happy, without adding in stress. You may have a few tweaks you wish to make to your new habits. All of these are good, and it means you are learning and finding ways to make it last for a lifetime.

Take it slow. Just as you didn't rush to start your detox, so you don't want to rush to come out of it. If you start eating heavier processed foods right away, drinking coffee and alcohol, or eating gluten, you are likely to have some digestive difficulties.

Your digestive system has been on a bit of a break and isn't used to digesting irritants. Take it slow. Add one thing back in at a time and see how you feel after consuming them. You may be surprised to notice that coffee or alcohol just doesn't seem as appealing or necessary anymore. You might notice that your previous intake of wheat and bread makes you feel bloated, gassy, and uncomfortable. These are all learning experiences and ways for you to see and incorporate what makes you feel good and what makes you feel not so good. Opt for the things that agree with your system and keep you feeling healthy and energized.

Remember, there is a reason you felt the need to start the detox program. There was something you were doing or a habit that you had that led you to cleanse. If you go right back to it, you'll be back in this same boat soon. Stick with some of the practices you've adopted during the previous 21 days and incorporate them when you can.

You have every tool within you to lead a vibrant life full of energy, fun, health, and satisfaction in every aspect. Here is your chance to take the lessons you learned and the tools you have and incorporate them into everyday life. Go forth. Stay healthy. Stay happy. And live the healthiest, happiest life that you deserve!

GROCERY LIST

From here on out, the way you decide to eat is completely up to you. Here is the challenge that I present to you: How did you feel during the cleanse? Cravings aside, did you feel healthier, happier, less stomach aches, more energy? If so, why go back to the foods that left you feeling less than optimal? With that thought in mind, you might decide to start adding in some of the items you refrained from during the detox. This is perfectly fine! Just see how they make you feel once you add them back in and stay open and aware of how your body and mind react to these items. If you decide to keep certain items out of your diet, try to think instead about all the foods you can have, rather than the ones you can't. It's all about adding in rather than taking away. This is what helps you not to feel deprived. Add in more vegetables and fruits, even if you start eating more meats, dairy, gluten, and sugars. If you stick to healthy veggies as a main part of your diet, you'll be well on your way to a healthy, happy you for life.

EXERCISE

As you move forward, keep exercising for at least 30 minutes every day. This can be broken up into short spurts throughout the day if necessary. It is just a way to break up sedentary moments and re-energize you - body, mind and spirit. Think of it not as just a workout, but as a way to keep your organs working smoothly, your digestive system on track, and your mind at peace. Remember, it doesn't have to be super intense. Do what you love, do what feels right for your body, and take some time to stretch and relax.

FOOD

It will be very tempting to head straight to the nearest store or restaurant and order anything on the menu you desire. In a few days you might go back to your previous eating habits and add in some of these foods, but starting that right away could lead to stomach upset and digestive problems. Since you haven't had specific ingredients in a while, adding them in all at once might make you feel sick. If you need to, slowly introduce them back one at a time each day, but see how you feel when you do. Give yourself a day or two between items such as sugar, meat, eggs, dairy, and gluten, as these can be the trigger for digestive intolerances, but might not show up right after you eat them. The important thing to remember when adding foods back in after your detox is this: You might feel good. You might feel not so good. Just remember to stay connected, present, and in tune with your body. This is the key to living the happy, healthy life you so very much deserve.

Chapter Ten: Recipes

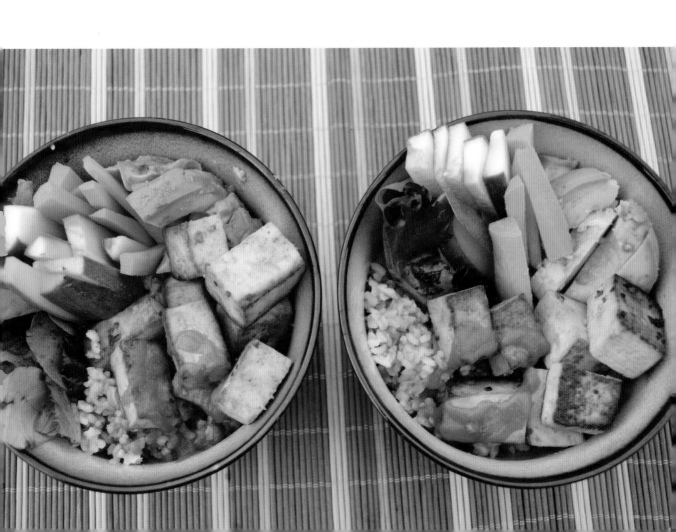

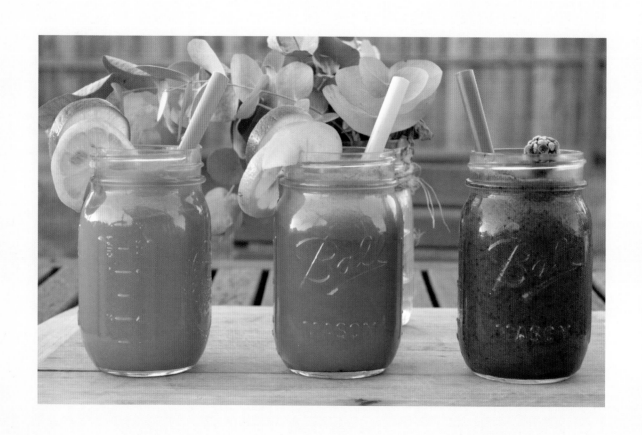

Juices and Smoothies

During your 21 day detox, you'll find that juices and smoothies become your lifeline and your new best friend. They pack a nutritional punch with each sip, are easy to make in a pinch, and leave you feeling energized and glowing from the inside out. Remember to keep them fresh and full of both fruit *and* green vegetables. The fruit adds a natural sweetness while the green vegetables keep it alkaline and super healthy for you.

Basic Green Juice

4 kale leaves
2 romaine leaves
1 handful spinach
1 handful mixed greens
1 large cucumber
1 lemon
1 apple (cored and deseeded)
*feel free to add any fresh herbs such as parsley, cilantro, mint, or basil to brighten up the flavors a little more

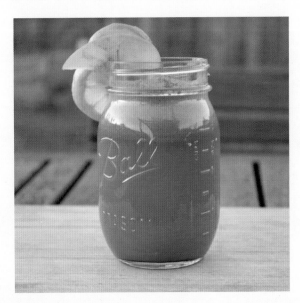

Start with the herbs and dark leafy greens (such as kale and spinach) and add them to the juicer. These have less water and create less juice. Then add the fruit and cucumber. These juicier items (a.k.a. cucumbers, apples, and lemons) help to push out the lingering juice from the juicer. Make sure to rinse your veggies first, keep the juicer running while adding items, and pour into a glass when finished.

Green and Clean Juice

1 cucumber

1 cup kale

1 cup spinach

1 apple or pear (cored and deseeded)

Juice of 1 lemon

Add all ingredients to your juicer, starting with the drier leafy greens first and working your way to the water rich cucumbers.

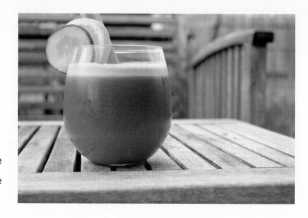

Green Zinger

1 cucumber

1 cup kale

1 cup spinach

1 inch of ginger

1 apple

1 lemon

Juice your leafy greens first, then your ginger, and finish with your fruit and cucumbers.

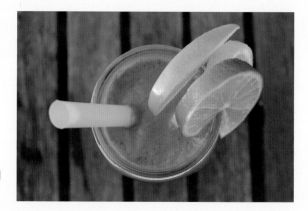

Root Veg Juice

Simply add each item into your juicer, starting with the leafier greens to the juicer ones. Pour into a glass and enjoy!

2 handfuls of spinach

5 leaves of kale

2 handfuls of mixed greens

2 celery stalks

1 large cucumber

2 apples (cored and deseeded)

Juice of 1 lime

1 large beet or 2 small beets

Optional: 1 piece of ginger (about ½ inch thick)

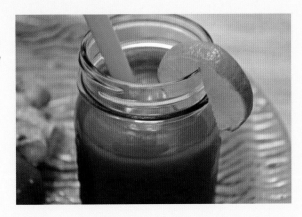

Juice your greens, root veggies, and fruit. Finish up with the cucumbers.

Detox Beet Juice

1 cup kale

1 cup spinach

1 inch ginger root

1 small beet

1 carrot

1 cucumber

1 apple (cored and deseeded)

Juice of 1 lime

Juice of 1 lemon

Add ingredients to your juicer, starting with the leafy greens and ginger first. Juice, drink, and enjoy!

Go Green Juice

1 to 2 lemons

¼ inch chunk ginger

handful of kale

2 apples

Add all ingredients into the juicer and enjoy!
It's green, detoxifying, hydrating, and tasty!

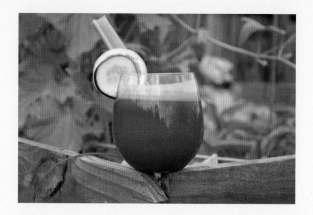

Sweet and Tangy Carrot Juice

3 large carrots

2 small apples (cored and deseeded)

1 large cucumber

Juice of 1 lemon

Juice of 1 lime

1 inch ginger

Add ingredients to juicer. Enjoy this juicy, tangy, sweet
drink.

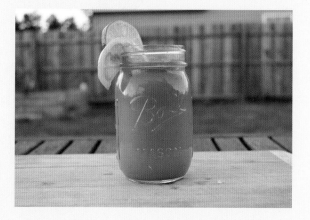

Cool Down Juice

1 cup kale

1 cup spinach

1 cucumber

1 cup watermelon

1 apple (cored and deseeded)

4 leaves romaine lettuce

1 sprig peppermint (optional)

1 lemon

Add ingredients to your juicer, starting with the leafy greens first, then add in the juicier items.

Green Lemonade

Makes one large juice.

2 apples (cored and deseeded)

Juice of 1 (large) lemon

1 cucumber

Juice in your juicer and enjoy!

Gorgeously Green Smoothie

1 cup kale

1 cup spinach

1 to 2 frozen bananas

½–1 cup vanilla coconut milk (unsweetened)

Add kale to the blender first and chop it up. Then add all other ingredients and blend until smooth. Pour into a cup and enjoy!

Strawberry Punch Juice

It's not only full of strawberry goodness; it is also great for digestion. Strawberry leaves, ginger, greens, and lemon are all digestive wonders when juiced.

1 to 2 cucumbers

Juice of 1 to 2 lemons

2–4 apples (cored and deseeded)

1 pint strawberries

1 inch ginger

2 handfuls spinach

Add all ingredients to the juicer, saving the cucumbers for last to push the rest of the juices through.

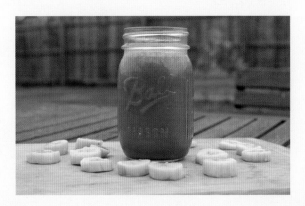

Green Detox Smoothie

1 cup kale

1 banana

½–1 freshly juiced apple juice (or plain non-dairy milk)

Juice of 1 lemon

Blend kale until chopped. Add in all other ingredients, adding in more liquid if needed, depending on the size of your fruit and speed of your blender.

Green and Clean Smoothie

1 cup spinach

1 cucumber (peeled)

1 apple (peeled and chopped)

½ avocado

½–1 cup water

Juice of 1 lemon

Blend spinach in your blender to chop it up. Add in other ingredients except lemon. Squeeze lemon juice into the smoothie and blend again until smooth.

Red Raspberry Smoothie

1 cup coconut milk or coconut water

1 cup fresh raspberries

1 frozen banana

2 tbsp chia seeds

Add all ingredients to your blender; turn it on and blend until smooth.

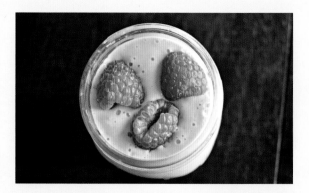

Blueberry Magic Smoothie

The base is green, but you would never know. It's like
magic! Makes 2 servings

1 cup frozen blueberries and/or blackberries

2 frozen bananas

1 cup unsweetened almond milk

2–3 handfuls of spinach

½ cucumber (peeled)

*optional natural liquid sweetener to taste

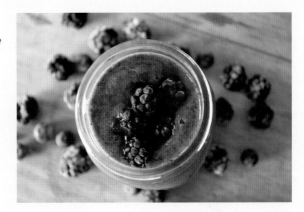

Blend all ingredients until smooth.

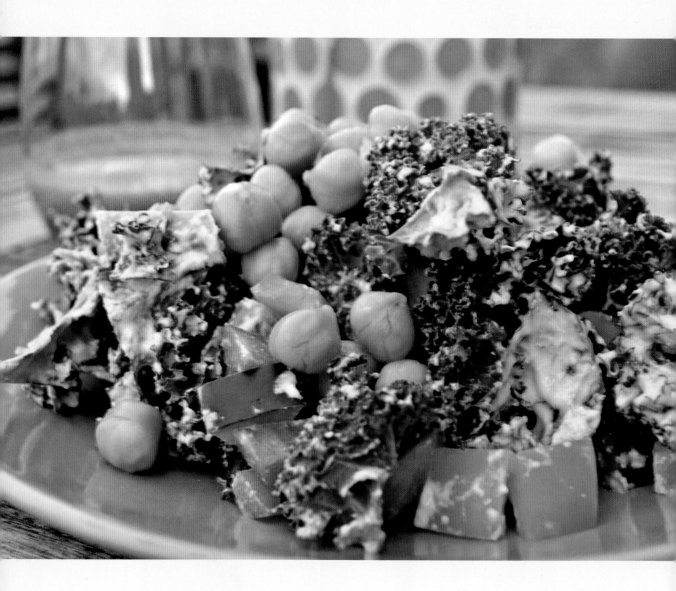

Salads and Soups

When you are trying to stay fresh and raw, soups and salads become a staple in your meal rotation. Add plenty of variety with fresh veggies, fruits, nuts, and seeds and you'll be sure to not get bored or feel deprived.

Carrot Ginger Soup

1 lb carrots

3 inches of ginger root, peeled and grated

1 to 2 cups coconut water

Peel and chop your carrots. Steam until soft. Add to a blender with ginger and coconut water. Start with 1 cup of coconut water and add more until you reach your desired thickness.

Butternut Squash Soup

1 butternut squash

1 tbsp coconut oil

1 large yellow onion, chopped

3 cloves garlic, diced

2 green onions, sliced

3 celery stalks, sliced

1 ½ cups filtered water

3 cups coconut milk, unsweetened, plain

1 tsp Himalayan sea salt

1 tsp black pepper

2 tbsp cinnamon

2 tsp nutmeg

1 tsp thyme

1 tsp rosemary

Peel the butternut squash and cut into chunks. Steam until soft. While steaming, heat coconut oil in a large sauté pan. Add in yellow onions, garlic, green onions, and celery. Cook until soft but not burnt. When cooked, add to a blender with 1 cup water. Blend until smooth. Once the squash in finished, remove it from the peel (either scoop or slice it away) and add it to the blender. Blend again until smooth. Add in coconut milk and spices (including salt and pepper). Blend once more. Adjust any spices as needed for your taste preference. If needed, heat again before serving. Otherwise, store in the refrigerator for and easy grab-n-go, nutrient packed meal!

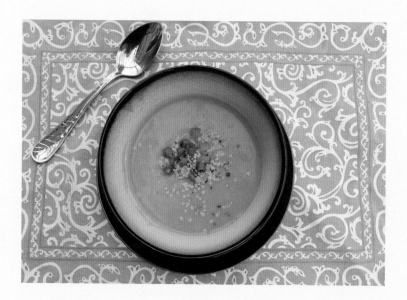

Taste the Rainbow Salad

You can change the veggies around for your liking, just remember the color wheel.

1 bunch romaine lettuce chopped

¼ red onion diced

1 carrot peeled and chopped

¼ head of broccoli, chopped

¼ bell pepper (green, red, yellow, or orange), diced

½ cucumber, chopped and deseeded if you prefer (keep the skins on though)

1 small tomato cut into 4 wedges

½ avocado, sliced

½ can chickpeas, rinsed and drained

1 piece sprouted grain bread, toasted in broiler and cut into pieces, for croutons

*sprouted grain bread contains higher amounts of protein and easier to digest carbohydrates, so you stay full longer without blood sugar spikes

Prepare all ingredients and pile high onto a plate or bowl. Top off with avocado, croutons, and dressing. It's as simple as that—everything you need for a complete meal on one plate.

Red and Blue Berry Salad

2 tbsp balsamic vinegar

1 tbsp grapeseed oil

pinch sea salt

½ tsp garlic powder

½ tsp Italian seasonings or oregano

Makes approximately 2 salads.

6 fresh strawberries, sliced

1 handful blueberries

2 tsp hemp seeds

½ cup almonds, sliced or chopped

1 large cucumber, chopped

2 cups/handfuls mixed greens

Whisk together vinegar, oil, salt, garlic powder, and seasonings. Add other ingredients into two bowls. Top with dressing.

Mango and Avocado Salad

Makes about 2 servings

½ mango, cubed

½ Avocado, cubed

¼ cucumber, cubed

⅛ onion, chopped

10 grape tomatoes, sliced in half

1 package of mixed greens (enough for 2 large servings)

¼ cup almond, pistachios, and/or cashews chopped in processor

2 tsp hemp seeds

The work is mostly in the prepping with this one! Pile all ingredients in a bowl. Top with Lemon-Tahini Dressing (recommended dressing for this one).

Detox Kale Salad

1 bunch/head of kale, stems removed

2 carrots, peeled and chopped

1 can chickpeas, drained and rinsed

½ yellow bell pepper, chopped

1 cucumber, peeled and chopped

Juice of 2 lemons, squeezed and juiced

3 tbsp tahini

1 tsp sea salt

1 to 2 tbsp water

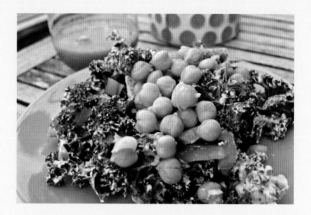

Remove kale stems and chop. Add all veggies and chickpeas into a bowl. In a blender, lemon juice, tahini, sea salt, and 1 tbsp of water. Blend until thick. If needed, add in more water. Remember you want this pretty thick but still able to pour.

Pour over the salad and mix thoroughly. Let it marinate for about 10 minutes and enjoy!

Dressings

A healthy salad dressing can be just the zing you need to take your salad from blah to unforgettably good.

Lemon Tahini Dressing

Makes enough for 2 to 3 salads

½ cup tahini

¼ cup water

Juice of 2 lemons (squeeze juice)

1 to 2 garlic cloves (or garlic powder if you're out of fresh garlic)

Salt to taste

Blend all ingredients in a blender until smooth. You want it pretty thin, the consistency of a salad dressing, but thicker than vinaigrette. Add more water if needed.

Basic Balsamic Vinaigrette

1 tbsp balsamic vinegar

2 tsp olive or grapeseed oil

Garlic powder, oregano, and sea salt to taste

Whisk all ingredients together and pour over salad

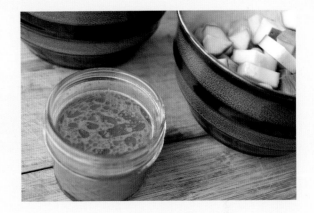

Honey Mustard Detox Vinaigrette

1 tbsp honey, agave, or pure maple syrup

2 tbsp mustard

Juice of ½ lemon, squeezed

½ tsp turmeric

½ tsp Himalayan sea salt

½ tsp black pepper

1 tsp apple cider vinegar

*optional 1 tsp freshly grated ginger

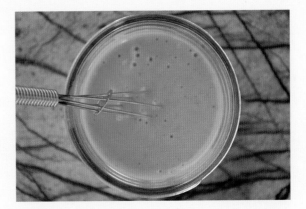

Whisk or blend all ingredients together. Pour over your salad.

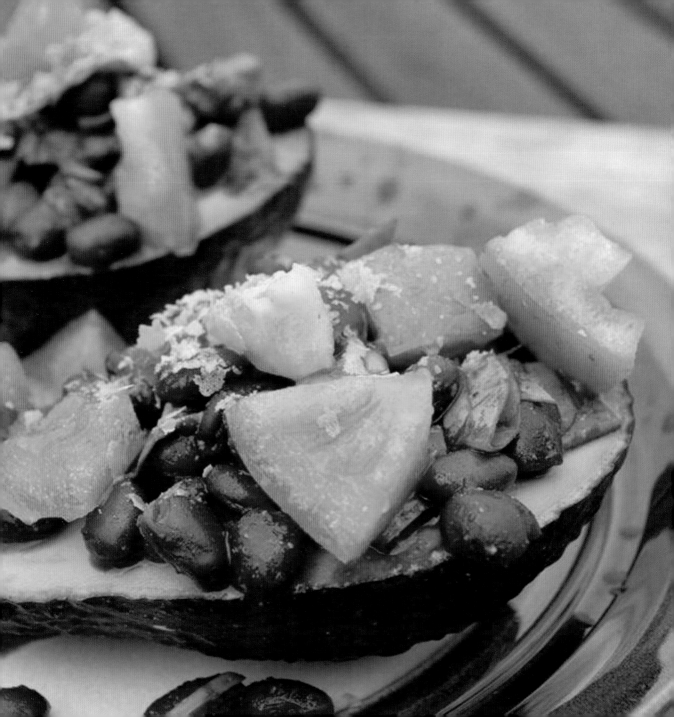

Lunches and Entrees

When you start eating healthy and experimenting with new foods and ingredients, you'll often be surprised at just how much variety you can add to your meals. These lunches and entrees are packed full of flavor and are simple to make. They heavy on the greens, which means each bite is packed with nutrients and vitamins. The recipes are easy to throw together. No complicated steps and no stress. Just healthy, delicious food you can make any time.

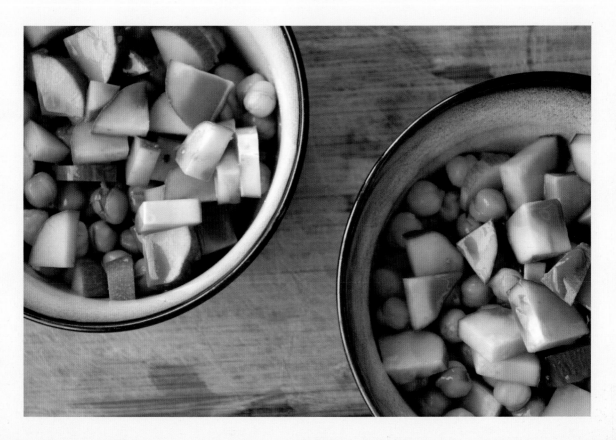

Mango Buddha Bowl

Makes 1 to 2 servings

½ to 1 cup brown rice

½ mango, cubed

¼ cucumber, cubed

⅛ onion, chopped

2 small red or orange bell peppers—the really tiny ones—or ½ one bell pepper, chopped

2 handfuls of kale, chopped, stems removed

1 to 2 tsp hemp seeds

1 tbsp chopped almonds, cashews, or pistachios

Lemon Tahini Dressing

Drop all ingredients into your bowl. Mix dressing thoroughly. Sprinkle with hemp seeds. Let sit for a minute to soften the kale and let the dressing seep in. Eat and enjoy.

Chickpea Taco Bowl with Homemade Seasoning

This serves about 2 to 3 people, depending on your portion sizes.

1 can chickpeas

juice of 1 lime (for juice)

¼ onion (your choice!)

Salsa as desired

2 to 3 tbsp chili powder

1 tsp cayenne

1 tsp paprika

½ tsp cumin

2 tbsp nutritional yeast

1 tsp salt (more or less as you prefer)

¼ cup water

1 to 2 cups cooked brown rice

1 avocado

4 leaves romaine lettuce

1 small tomato

Drain and rinse can of chickpeas. Pulse in a blender until lightly chopped – leave them in a "crumbled meat" texture. Place in a pan on the stove over medium heat. Add seasonings and water. Stir together until incorporated. Adjust seasonings as needed. Cook until heated through, about 5 minutes. Place in a bowl over the rice and top with avocado, salsa, tomatoes, onions, and any other veggies you like!

Black Bean Buddha Bowl

Makes 2 servings

2 cups cooked brown rice

1 can black beans, drained and rinsed

1 red bell pepper, chopped

2 cups spinach, chopped

1 avocado

1 small tomato

1 tsp garlic powder

1 tbsp chili powder

1 tbsp nutritional yeast

1 tsp cayenne powder

1 tbsp water

pinch of sea salt

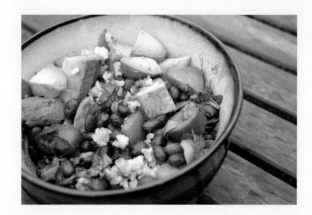

Drain and rinse the black beans. In a pot, add beans, salt, nutritional yeast, and spices on medium high heat. Add in the water and stir until heated and mixed together thoroughly. In two bowls, add the beans, rice, spinach, peppers, tomato, and avocado.

Brussels Sprouts and Tofu Bowl

10 Brussels sprouts, cut in half

2 servings of brown rice

1 block firm tofu, pressed and drained

2 tbsp coconut oil

2 tbsp reduced-sodium tamari

2 tsp sesame seeds

1 tbsp agave nectar (or, if you eat honey that will work too)

2 tsp garlic powder

Cook the brown rice according to package directions. Feel free to season it with sesame seeds/oil, coconut oil, or garlic powder as desired.

Drain your tofu, wrap it in a paper towel and place between two plates. Rest a heavy object on top and let it squeeze out the moisture for at least 20 minutes, preferably longer. You want the tofu firm and dry, so that it will soak up your marinade.

Once pressed, cut the tofu into cubes and place in a container with agave nectar, 1 tbsp tamari, 1 tsp garlic powder, and 1 tsp sesame seeds. Shake well to coat the tofu and let it sit for about 20 minutes or longer again.

While the tofu is marinating, cut your Brussels sprouts in half and heat a pan with the remaining coconut oil. Add the sprouts to the pan over medium-high heat. Cook until browned and flip over. You want them to get crispy and remain a little firm. Once you flip them, add the rest of the garlic powder and tamari to the pan. If needed, you can add extra tamari. Add in the tofu and brown the sides to get crispy. Once everything is cooked through, remove from the pan.

Scoop you rice into two bowls and serve your Brussels sprouts and tofu on top.

Simple Sautéed Brussels Sprouts

1 bag/package of fresh Brussels sprouts

Sea salt, black pepper, rosemary, and garlic powder to taste

1 tbsp olive oil to drizzle

Heat oil in sauté pan on medium-high heat.

Slice Brussels sprouts in half. Place face down in a sauté pan. Sprinkle the seasonings into your pan and cover with a lid. After 2 to 3 minutes, flip and brown the back side of the Brussels sprouts. Heat for an additional 2 minutes until browned but firm.

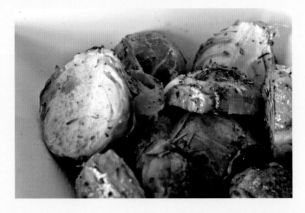

Spicy Kale and Tomatoes

2 cups kale, chopped and stems removed

½ cup cherry or grape tomatoes, cut in half

1 to 2 tsp olive oil (in pan)

1 tsp nutritional yeast, sprinkled

1 tsp cayenne powder

2 tsp garlic powder

1 pinch sea salt

1 tsp turmeric

Heat olive oil in your pan over high heat. Reduce to medium heat and add your kale. Toss gently. After 1 minute, add you tomatoes and seasonings. Continue cooking for 1 to 2 more minutes.

Serve with your favorite whole, gluten-free grains and enjoy!

Black Bean Stuffed Avocado

1 avocado, sliced in half, seed removed

½ can of black beans

½ to 1 small tomato, chopped

1 handful spinach, chopped

2 tsp chili powder

2 tsp garlic powder

1 tsp cumin

½ tsp cayenne

½ tsp curry

Salt to taste

2 tbsp water

Nutritional yeast

Drain and rinse black beans. Heat over medium high heat. Add in spices and water. Stir until heated all the way through. When finished cooking, scoop into avocados, where the seed used to be. Top with nutritional yeast, spinach, and tomatoes.

Tempeh Scramble

Makes enough for 2 servings

1 package of tempeh, cut into cubes
1 small green bell pepper
¼ to ½ sweet onion
1 cup spinach, chopped
¼ cup water
Olive oil for pan (about 1 to 2 tsp)
Turmeric, nutritional yeast, garlic, and sea salt to taste

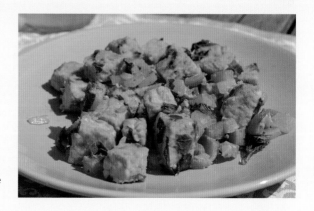

Chop onions, peppers and spinach. Heat olive oil over medium-high heat. Add tempeh to the pan. Cook for about 2 minutes. Then add onions and peppers. Cook for another 2 minutes. Add spices and water. Cook an additional minute tor two.

Balsamic Cucumber and Beet Bowl

Makes 1 Bowl

1 can chickpeas, drained and rinsed
1 beet, peeled, chopped
1 cup spinach
2 tbsp balsamic vinegar
1 pinch sea salt

Steam beets until soft. While steaming, prepare chickpeas and chop spinach. When the beets are cooked, add all ingredients to a bowl and mix together.

Chickpea Cucumber Salad:

1 can chickpeas, rinsed and drained
½ cucumber, de-seeded and chopped
⅛ onion (just a tbsp or so) chopped
Balsamic Vinegar to drizzle

Open can. Drain and rinse. Chop veggies. Assemble into a bowl. Drizzle on desired amount of vinegar. Mix together and eat. Lunch in less than 5 minutes.

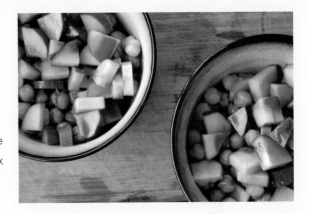

Coconut Sweet Potato Fries:

So easy. So tasty. So good for you.
1 sweet potato, peeled
1 tsp coconut oil
Himalayan sea salt to sprinkle

Slice sweet potatoes into ¼ inch thick, 1 inch wide strips. Coat pan lightly with coconut oil and heat over medium-high heat. Place sweet potatoes in pan. Sprinkle lightly with sea salt.
Allow to cook for 2 to 3 minutes. Flip, sprinkle lightly with sea salt, and cook on this side for 2 to 3 minutes. Repeat on all four sides (as much as possible).
Serve and enjoy! These fries are light, tasty, with a hint of coconut.

Simple Greens

2 cups chopped kale (other greens work well too), stems removed
1 tsp olive oil
1 tbsp nutritional yeast
1 tsp turmeric
Sea salt and garlic powder to taste

Heat olive oil on high. Add kale and seasonings. Cook until the kale is wilted and brightens in color. Serve and enjoy!

Spicy Tofu Bowls for Two:

This is one of my favorite meals. Feel free to play with the ingredients and add your own favorite combinations!

2 tbsp sriracha hot sauce

1 tsp agave nectar

1 tbsp tamari

1 tsp coconut oil

1 tsp ground ginger

1 tsp garlic powder

2 tsp sesame seeds

½ to 1 package pressed, drained tofu

1 package mixed greens

1 avocado, sliced

1 carrot, peeled and chopped

1 cucumber, peeled and chopped

¼ red onion, diced

2 cups cooked Brown Rice

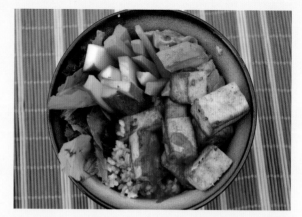

Cook the rice, either ahead of time or before you start to prepare the rest of the meal, as it takes the longest to cook. While the rice is cooking, press your tofu. Drain the water out of the package. Place on a plate, wrapped in a paper towel, if you have them. Place another plate on top. Top this with a heavy book or object. Let it press/drain for 30 minutes. Remove the towels and drain the water. Cut into cubes.

While the tofu is pressing, you can start your marinade. Add the ground ginger, garlic powder, agave, 1 tsp of tamari, 1 tsp of sriracha to a large bowl. Whisk all ingredients together. Add tofu cubes and marinate for another 20 minutes. By this time, the rice should be finished.

Heat coconut oil on the stove in a sauté pan on medium heat. When it melts/heats, add the marinated tofu. Heat until browned/blackened on one side, then flip and brown the other side. In your bowls you will eat out of, assemble your ingredients: rice, then mixed greens, then tofu. Top with ½ avocado, ½ of the diced onions, ½ carrot, and ½ cucumber. Use the rest of the tamari and the sriracha as your dressing. Sprinkle with sesame seeds as desired.

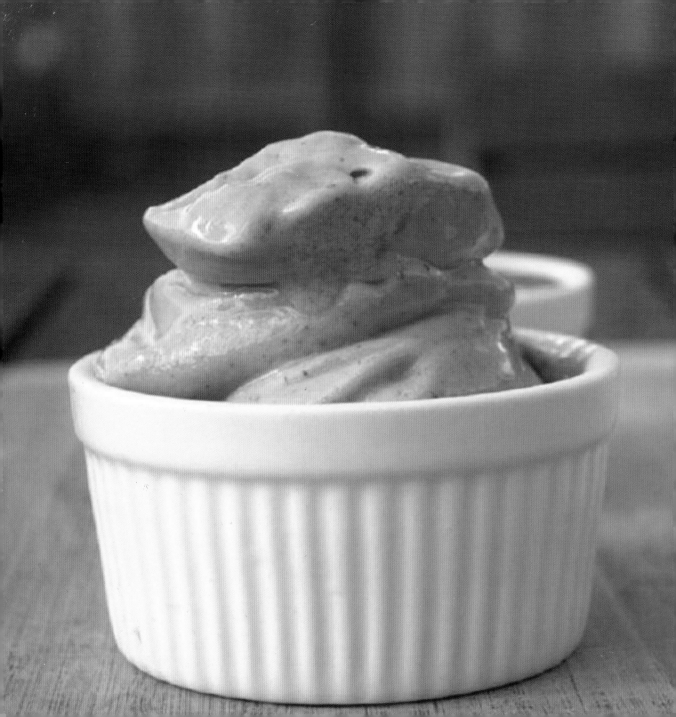

DESSERTS, SNACKS, BARS, AND BREAKFASTS

What you eat in the middle of your day and between meals can often make or break your cleanse. Eat too much and you'll reverse much of the work you've done. Eat too little and you'll crash and burn before the day is over. Enjoy a healthy snack in between meals when needed, just keep it clean, whole, and pure.

Almond Butter Dates

4 Medjool Dates (the big ones), pitted and cut in half lengthwise
1 to 2 tbsp almond butter
2 tsp hemp seeds

Stuff date halves with almond butter. Sprinkle with hemp seeds. Eat and smile or refrigerate until later.

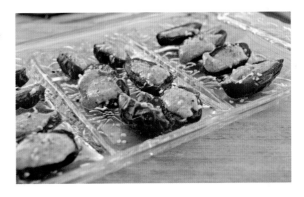

Simple Detox Tea

Don't let the color scare you! Turmeric turns things a deep yellow color.
½ tsp Turmeric
Juice of ½ Lemon, squeezed
½ tsp Cayenne
1 tsp Honey (optional)

Boil water. Place ingredients in mug. Add hot/warm water. Stir. If it's not too hot, sip, smile, and enjoy!

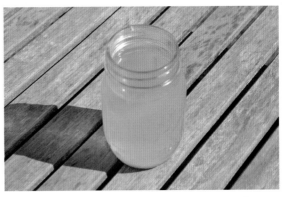

Berry Ice Cream

1 cup frozen berries (any kind)

¼ cup coconut cream or milk

Agave nectar or natural sweetener to taste

Add all ingredients to a blender. Blend until thick and scoopable, but not chunky, like ice cream. Add more blueberries or creamer to reach desired consistency. Taste and blend with sweetener if needed, it all depends on your taste buds and the blueberries!

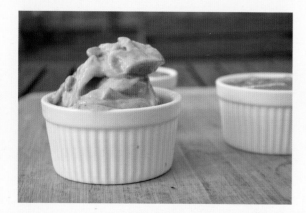

Banana Soft Serve

1 cup berries

1 frozen banana

½ tbsp Agave nectar, honey, or maple syrup if needed

Add all ingredients to your blender and process until smooth. You can stop to scrape the sides if needed.

Vanilla Vegan Overnight Oats

½ cup oats

1tsp ground flax seeds

1tsp chia seeds

1 tsp hemp seeds

1 cup (approximately) vanilla coconut milk (or any that you choose)

Place all dry ingredients in a mason jar. Add milk until it almost fills the jar. Stir together. Don't worry if it seems thin, it will thicken up fast! Place in fridge with lid on overnight.

In the morning, open, grab a spoon, and top with fresh berries!

Coconut Popcorn

1 to 2 tbsp coconut oil

¼ cup popcorn kernels

sprinkle of (Himalayan) sea salt

*you'll also need a large pot—not too heavy, a lid, and a few pot holders

Heat oil on high. Add in kernels. Cover with lid. When they start popping, grab the potholders and start shaking the pot back and forth over the burner - this helps to get to all the kernels and keeps the popped ones from burning. Continue until you hear no more popping.

Carrot and Date Bowl

Makes 2 to 3 servings

6 large organic carrots

1 tbsp organic coconut oil

10 dates

2 tbsp organic hemp seeds (shelled). Steam the carrots until soft. When they are cooked, add carrots and coconut oil to a high-powered blender. Blend until fully pureed.

Scoop into bowls. Top with dates and sprinkle with hemp seed.

Eat and enjoy!

Homemade Raw Almond Butter

1 lb raw almonds

Blend in a food processor for approximately 15 minutes until smooth, creamy, and a bit drippy. You may need to pause the processor to scrape the sides several times.

Apple Cinnamon Energy Bars

1 cup raw almonds, soaked for 20 minutes

1 dehydrated apple, or 1 package dried apple slices (soft)

10 pitted dates

1 to 2 tsp cinnamon (to taste)

If you are dehydrating your own apple—cut into thin rings and dehydrate approximately 6 hours until the rings are slightly hard. *You can also use store bought dried apple slices if you don't own a dehydrator or are short on time. Just look for one with minimal to no preservatives.*

Soak almonds in a bowl of water for at least 20 minutes to soften. After 20 minutes and after apples are dehydrated, add all ingredients into a high speed blender or food processor. Blend until incorporated, but allow the almonds to stay a bit chunky.

Spread onto a piece of parchment paper. Top with another piece and roll out into a square shape. You can also press into a bread pan if available. Transfer into a freezer safe pan and press top flat. Remove top piece of parchment. Cut into 1 inch thick pieces (lengthwise). Place in freezer for about 1 hour, until firm. Transfer to individual bags or containers and store in fridge until ready to grab-n-go!

Superfood Chocolate Protein Bars

Makes approximately 10 bars, give or take a few depending in your cutting size.

¼ cup dark chocolate powder

½ cup ground flax seed

2 tbsp chia seed

½ tsp spirulina

½ cup almond butter

2 ½ cups oatmeal, blended

½ cup agave nectar (or natural sweetener of choice)

¾ cup hot water

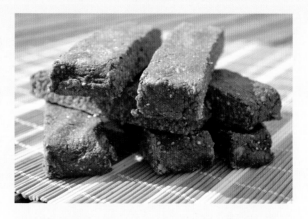

Blend oatmeal until it is almost flour-like in consistency, but still a bit chunky. Mix all ingredients, except water, together in a bowl. You may need to get in there with your hands to really incorporate it all together. Slowly add water in small amounts. You want your mixture slightly wet so it can clump together, but not runny.

In a parchment paper-lined casserole dish, spread your mixture out evenly. Refrigerate for 1 hour. Cut into 10 bars or any other shape you would like. Keep refrigerated until ready to eat.

Energy Balls

⅔ cup cashews

¾ cup oats (for gluten free, use certified GF oats)

Pinch of Himalayan Sea Salt

7 pitted dates, chopped

1 tsp pure vanilla extract

4 tbsp agave nectar

1 tbsp molasses

3 to 4 tbsp dark chocolate (chips or chunks)

Mix cashews and oats together in a food processor. Combine until flour-like in texture. Add salt and dates, mix for 1 minute. Add vanilla, agave, and molasses. Mix until the dough becomes sticky and almost combined together. Add in chocolate and process for 10 seconds. Scoop with hands and roll into small dough balls. Place on a greased tray or parchment paper. Place in freezer for one hour and enjoy!

RESOURCES AND INFORMATION:

The House of Healthy: thehouseofhealthy.com

The Institute for Integrative Nutrition Book: integrativenutriton.com

Crazy, Sexy, Diet, by Kris Carr: Kriscarr.com

Diet for a New America, by John Robbins: johnrobbins.info

The Chopra Center: chopra.com

The Himalayan Institute: himalayaninstitute.org

The Hippocrates Institute: hippocratesinst.org

Forks over Knives Documentary: Forksoverknives.com

Environmental Working Group: EWG.com

Fat, Sick, and Nearly Dead Documentary: rebootwithjoe.com

Gluten-Free Diet/Lifestyle: glutenfree.com

Dr. Joel Fuhrman: drfuhrman.com

Dr. Neal Barnard: nealbarnard.org

Dr. Mark Hyman: drhyman.com

Dr. Andrew Weil: drweil.com

ABOUT THE AUTHOR

Jessi Andricks is a certified Yoga teacher, Health Coach, mind-body fitness instructor and writer living just outside Charleston, SC. Jessi has been featured on multiple health and wellness sites, including My Yoga Online, Book Yoga Retreats, Chic Vegan, and Yoga Download. Her recipes have even been awarded the designation of "Best Appetizer Recipe Ever" on the BetterRecipes.com blog, The Daily Dish. She has trained in Health Coaching, Ayurveda, Green Living, and multiple mind-body fitness formats. Jessi lives her passion for a healthy life by teaching and inspiring others through empowering yoga classes, juicing and detox workshops, and a love for an energetic life. Jessi lives by her truth—we all have the tools within us to live the healthy, happy lives we deserve. You can find more from Jessi at www.thehouseofhealthy.com.

INDEX